Breast Cancer

A Soul Journey

Breast Cancer

A Soul Journey

Patricia Greer

CHIRON PUBLICATIONS
ASHEVILLE, NORTH CAROLINA

Book and cover design by Marianne Jankowski.
Cover photograph by Patricia Greer.
Printed in the United States of America.

Library of Congress Cataloging-in-Publication Data

Greer, Patricia, 1940-
Breast cancer : a soul journey / Patricia Greer.
pages cm
Includes bibliographical references and index.
ISBN 978-1-63051-087-9 (pbk. : alk. paper) -- ISBN 978-1-63051 088-6 (hardcover : alk. paper)
1. Greer, Patricia, 1940---Health. 2. Breast--Cancer--Patients--United States--Biography. 3. Breast--Cancer--Psychological aspects. I. Title.

RC280.B8G724 2014
616.99'4490092--dc23
[B]

2014032387

To the women of the sisterhood

and to all who hear and honor

the whispers of soul

Put your ear down close to your soul and listen hard.

—Anne Sexton

CONTENTS

PREFACE

I remember exactly where I was when the call came. My husband and I were having an early dinner at the kitchen table when the phone rang; I answered and heard my surgeon tell me I had breast cancer. I stared out the window at a bleak February evening while he carefully explained the treatment options available to me, but I didn't hear much of what he said after the words "breast cancer."

The experience of having breast cancer was paradoxically the most alienating and the most connecting one of my life. I felt deeply and existentially alone as I faced the next six months of surgery, chemotherapy, and radiation; this was my path to walk. And yet I also felt more intensely and authentically connected to my family and close friends, whom I knew would walk with me.

In the early days of treatment, I spoke on the phone with a woman named Linda who was undergoing breast cancer treatment at the same hospital. She had volunteered to talk to other women with the disease, and the oncology staff had given me her name. I had many questions for her, but even more important than her answers were the opportunities to laugh together about wanting pizza and wine and chocolate after chemotherapy and to cry together about losing our hair.

I never got to meet Linda. She died before we were able to connect in person, and I never had the chance to tell her how much those early moments of sharing meant to me. She had given me a lifeline when I most needed it, and I am forever grateful to her. I thank her for her help, her compassion and humor and bravery, and I hope my words may reach out to others, as hers did to me, with some measure of hope and healing power and potential for growth.

Since the illness, I have felt a strong bond with other women who have had breast cancer. I sometimes imagine us as an army of women who are fighting like the soldiers of the past who lined up for combat in full view of the enemy. In this battle, we stand together as warriors and face the common adversary; when one falls, another takes her place in the fight. On a literal level, we are each fighting the disease, and we must support each other as comrades do. But perhaps there are other adversaries we also need to identify and confront. As women, do we share some common enemies, either external or internal? As a sisterhood, do we have common issues we need to address?

These pages are an invitation to women with breast cancer to explore possible meanings and messages of the disease. As a Jungian analyst, I am interested in working with metaphor and exploring the inner meanings of experiences. I share my exploration of the images and meanings associated with my experience of the disease in the hope that it may offer examples for other women who want to reflect on their experiences and find insights and lessons that may be gained from viewing cancer as a teacher.

Some women may not feel called to take this kind of journey; they may believe that for them the best way of dealing with the illness is to put it behind them and move on. There is no right or wrong way of responding; each individual knows what is best for her. For women who do want to explore their experience of breast cancer, seeking the wisdom embedded in it, this book offers one possible map. My associations and meanings are personal but many resonate with other women giving voice to similar concerns. I have used my own images, dreams, inner journeys, and poetry as examples of ways of deepening into and under the reality of cancer. I have collected excerpts from poets, philosophers, and psychologists to illuminate the way, and I have collected words from women who are addressing feminine questions and concerns connected with my own.

There are many crises that can interrupt a life, wake us up, demand that we pay more attention to the way we are living. Breast cancer has been such a summons for me and for many other women. These pages offer ways of thinking about metaphor and ways of exploring the meanings of breast cancer. The answers will be unique to each person who goes through the experience, but perhaps we can all share in the struggle to learn from cancer, to understand more about ourselves, to become more fully ourselves. Perhaps it can be, for each of us, a soul journey.

ACKNOWLEDGMENTS

My appreciation . . .

To my husband, Carl, who walked with me through my journey with breast cancer and my soul journey of exploration, who supported my healing and writing. He encouraged me to be wherever I needed to be and was there with me and for me . . .

To my children, Mike, Susie, and Jeannie, my good friends, who shared my fears and hopes, my tears and laughter . . .

To my friends and family and colleagues, who helped me get through the tough times. To Nancy, who came when I needed her. To Linda and Cynthia and Vivian and Patty, who hung in with me through it all. To Carolyn and Dee and Pam, who envisioned healing. To Becky, who saw with wisdom. To Judi and Marty, who cared up close. To Peg and Joyce, who cared from afar. To Barbara and Nancy, who helped me come home to bodysoul. To Dianne and Olga, who encouraged me in the process. To Diane, who trusted the rhythms of psyche even when I did not. To Joanie, who joined me in the search and helped me remember to love to write. To my parents, who expressed their love and concern. To my sister, Sue, who always let me know that she cared . . .

To the early readers of this book. To my husband, who read and discussed many versions and who is my strongest advocate. To my children, who gave me good suggestions and lots of encouragement. To my friends and colleagues Linda, Cynthia, Judi, Ellen, Julia, and Jeannie, who all offered insights and perspectives that helped me craft a better book . . .

To my editor, Elizabeth Eowyn Nelson, author and teacher, who was instrumental in making this book a reality. She is fluent in the language of soul work and was a delight to work with. . .

To all the folks at Chiron Publications, especially Len Cruz and Steve Buser, who welcomed me with enthusiasm, and to Siobhan Drummond, editor and producer, who worked with my manuscript with care and respect . . .

To my clients, who have trusted me to accompany them on parts of their soul journeys and from whom I have learned much . . .

To all my teachers throughout the years . . .

And to Gram, who blessed me early in my life with the poet's words, "Homeward serenely she walked with God's benediction upon her" . . .

. . . with gratitude and love

1

Metaphor and Meaning

Consciousness will not always solve the problem, but it may make the suffering meaningful.

—Marion Woodman, *The Owl Was a Baker's Daughter*

BREAST CANCER. For most women, the words carry deep and devastating fear: fear of the disfigurement or loss of a breast and all it may represent, fear of the ordeal of treatment, and fear, ultimately, of death. My own confrontation with breast cancer began twenty-six years ago when I was forty-seven. It felt, as it does for many women, as if my life was ripped apart: there was life before cancer and there would be life, I hoped, after cancer. But there was a deep and essential difference between the two.

There is a painting by Georgia O'Keeffe titled *Abstraction, Blue* which captures my experience most vividly. It is strong and graceful, feminine in its rounded shapes and curves. The painting is done in swirls of color, mostly blues and greens, with a whisper of pale pink near the top and deepening layers of black toward the bottom. Slashed through the center is a fissure, a crevice, as if the painting had been sliced apart and the two sides moved, slightly crookedly, away from each other, never again to fit quite so neatly together. Without the gap, the painting might be too pretty: soft shapes, movement, gentle tones played in harmony, pleasing to the eye. But there is that gash right through the middle of the piece, creating a space and a tension.

This painting carries much of the image of breast cancer for me, in both its destructive and life-giving aspects. The feminine curves, breastlike and womanly, are asymmetrical and don't quite fit together. The whole picture is off a little, like seams in the wallpaper that don't quite match. That's the way life felt to me: off-kilter, not matched, never again to be a seamless whole, never again to be so simple.

As I began the journey to make meaning of my experience, I came across words written by Annie Dillard. Her description of the "gap through which eternity streams" was a powerful affirmation of the potential growth that can come from such a rupture.[1] Life which is too closed, too self-contained and satisfied and apparently whole, leaves no room for the piercing intensity of the appearance of something larger. One has to feel torn open to allow such entrance.

Externally, I dealt with the realities of the cancer growth: I had surgery to remove the malignant lump in my breast, followed by radiation and chemotherapy to attempt to eradicate any other cancer cells in my body. The medical procedures were powerful and effective; in spite of several incidents of suspected relapse, I have not yet had a recurrence of the disease.

I remember one of my early chemotherapy treatments. My husband sat with me as I reclined in a chair and had an intravenous infusion of the drugs that would hopefully save my life. As we exited the hospital after the session, I saw our favorite Italian restaurant across the street and wanted to go there for dinner. Groggy from the medications, I could barely walk straight; my husband wisely talked me out of the three-cheese lasagna I craved and got me home before the nausea struck. And then he had to deal with my requests for chocolate pudding and cake in between periods of vomiting. In time, my oncologist was able to adjust the combination of drugs so that I experienced less nausea, but there were other difficult realities to endure over the six months of chemotherapy: the major side effects of hair loss and fatigue and the minor problems of skin rashes and mouth sores.

And there were also emotional realities to endure. Although the cure rate for breast cancer is relatively high, depending on the size and stage of the tumor, I had to confront death in a close and personal way. The shadow of fear never goes away. Every ache, every twinge, every physical symptom brings an immediate reaction of alarm and apprehension that the cancer has returned. Life is terminal, and I was forced to face this realization again and again, in ways I'd never had to before.

Every mammogram brings with it a specter of death. I remember sitting in waiting rooms with groups of women gathered to have the tests that would indicate whether or not we had breast cancer. We never spoke with each other, perhaps in recognition of the intensity of the moment or the deep need for privacy in this solitary challenge. Was anyone praying? I don't know about the others; I was.

I felt the presence of death at those times, both a fear of actual death and an awareness of a kind of deadening of my spirit. Did I have to deaden parts of myself to endure this procedure? Was I afraid that repeated exposure to the fear of death was itself deadening? I remember the words I wrote about the experience:

> I wait in the room
> while they look at the black pictures
> to see if the cancer is there
> still
> or again.

I look out across city space
at the buildings,
rows and rows of windows
like hundreds of dead eyes,
hiding any secrets of life,
only mirroring.

I feel a part of me dead:
not only where the lump
grew
but other parts of me too
which hide the life
and only mirror.

A mirror is hard and flat.
A person
should not be.

Dead eyes
and black pictures
and mirrors.
And me.

In addition to the medical interventions of surgery, chemotherapy, and radiation, I also relied on the spiritual practices of prayer and meditation and used guided imagery to envision the dynamics of what was going on inside my body. I wanted to enlist strong but nonviolent inner allies, so I imagined the cancer cells being surrounded and safely carried away by my inner helpers. When I received chemotherapy, I thought of it not as poison, as some have called it, but as a forceful antidote to the out-of-control cancer cells. When I received radiation, I pictured calm colors of blue and green flowing through my body with healing potential. I believe in the power of the mind-body link, and although I didn't understand all the complex interactions, I wanted to engage all the help I could summon.

But the most powerful and important aspect of my work with cancer is, I believe, the psychological dimension of exploration through image, through metaphor and symbol. This is the spiritual and psychological growth that has come from the opening which cancer provided. From unwanted cancer growth came growth of soul for me. This is a different kind of imaginal work, not focused on curing the disease, although it may have some effect on the course of the illness. Rather, it is about a metaphorical encircling of the lump which allows for the richness of a different kind of growth. It is not about eradicating the symptom, but about searching for meaning and depth in the experience. It is a healing in search of *wholing*, of becoming more whole, of becoming more fully oneself.

I have worked with the symptom and the symbol of cancer, the sense of growth that is out of control and growth that may be pushing for birth. I have worked with the image of the mothering breast, of issues with my own mother, with the mother figure within, with the mother I have been and am. I have worked with issues of feeding and nurturing, with difficult choices about giving and withholding. I have worked with the rock-hard rage against the patriarchal oppression of women and the stone of silence closing off expression. I have worked with the image of a lump that grows like a knot close to my heart, of a lump as a weight, pulling me into the matter of my body, deepening me into the wisdom of cell energy. I have worked with the lump that grew hidden in my body, becoming the secret around which my soul grew, the irritation that was transformed into a pearl. And I have begun to learn of the spiraling journey around and toward soul.

I don't think there is a right way to deal with breast cancer. I didn't write at all for a year after I received the diagnosis. And then, almost exactly a year later, I began to write again, to keep a journal, to explore the symbolic meanings of my own inner experience. Perhaps I needed a year of mourning all the losses, or perhaps I just needed all my energy to live through the physical and emotional ordeal.

The meanings and associations I have discovered on my journey with breast cancer have been invaluable. They have made it possible for me to live with the shadow of the disease and to live richly not only in spite of, but because of, the threat of cancer. I don't intend to romanticize the ordeal of breast cancer; there are grim and terrible realities to face, and eventually the specter of death. But I have also found that cancer can be life-enhancing and soul-enriching. My focus is not to deny the physical fact but to add to it the richness of meaning found in an exploration of imaginal layers of reality, of metaphors and meanings encircling the lump of cancer.

To work with the meaning of illness is to seek the symbol within the disease, to see if the illness might be calling us to make adjustments in our attitudes, our perspectives, our lives. Carl Jung said, "the gods have become diseases."[2] To speak of the gods in this way is to move into the world of the metaphorical. Such gods are not to be understood as literal retaliatory deities who cause disease as punishment for sin or wrongdoing. Rather, they are personifications of universal energies or aspects of personality; they are inner figures in the soul's search for wholeness and individuation, the lifelong process of becoming more fully oneself. The gods of psyche, carrying such demands for becoming whole, may speak through illness.

I found other writers who share this view. Russell Lockhart writes of the presence of such gods when he suggests that we understand illness as a wounding; we need to seek out and connect with the god hidden there, an aspect of oneself which has been disregarded, dishonored. He believes connecting with the god within the symptom, within the illness, means connecting with the denied possibilities within oneself. Lockhart envisions cancer as the feared other that can destroy but can also trigger a process of inner growth leading to the creation of a greater personality. It may challenge us to confront the ultimate meaning and purpose of our destiny.[3]

Albert Kreinheder also speaks of the value of illness as an opportunity for growth and believes it can lead us to a reconnection with "our center and source," a sense of homecoming. He suggests disease has symbolic content, which "enters the soul through the wound of the body" and sets up a struggle in which one may "grow beyond one's former boundaries."[4]

Some critics believe such an exploration of meaning in the experience of cancer blames and shames the patient. They feel that if we are open to the view of cancer as a teacher, as a way of summoning us to new possibilities in our lives, then we, the cancer patients, must have been doing something "wrong" which caused the cancer. I think we need to distinguish between meaning and cause. We don't know all the factors that may contribute to cancer; I am not interested in determining cause but in exploring meaning which may lead to transformation. Perhaps we can look within the illness to see what we may be called to become, without suggesting a causal relationship.

There are many ways of approaching the idea of the meaning and metaphor of breast cancer. My own exploration is about a particular kind of meaning, the metaphorical and symbolic exploration of the idea and experience of breast cancer as it resonated in my psyche and in my life. This orientation moves outside of the issues of causality, blame, and healing. I do believe in the intricate and intimate relationship of psyche and body and the possibility that psychological realities can activate healing. I also believe that healing is not the same as cure, that healing of the soul may be more essential than cure of the body, and that the symptom of an illness may need to be understood as a call for a shift in consciousness.

My work with imagery is an attempt to allow psyche to express itself and to facilitate a dialogue with unknown parts of myself. This is an exploration of the inner landscape populated by the vistas and figures of psyche calling for attention, for honoring, for change. It is a nonlinear journey, a circling around the reality and metaphor of cancer, allowing meanings to appear and shift and transform. It involves a meandering energy which can spiral and deepen.

To move into this world, we need to create a sense of sacred space, an inner sanctuary where images can be held and honored. One of the first experiences I had with cancer was a sense of clearing out interior space and of valuing the richness of the emptiness. As I continued my journey, I practiced an indwelling awareness and focused intensely on the image of cancer as metaphor, using several methods to deepen my exploration, including keeping a journal, writing poetry, practicing active imagination, drawing, doing sand tray work, and paying attention to dreams. All these methods help to access the deeper levels of oneself. Working with dreams and sometimes drawing them or seeing what appears in the sand tray are all ways of using active imagination to allow aspects of the unconscious to appear. Drawing, painting, or writing about an image can sometimes lead to surprising details not seen or known before.

Writing is one of the primary ways in which I connect with deeper parts of myself; whether it is keeping a journal or composing prose or poetry, the written word takes me to another way of knowing.

> I write to know.
> It's as if I don't know
> until the words come,
> until the words tell me what I know.

It's not to remember, exactly,
it doesn't feel like that,
although somewhere I know
before words.

I write to see,
to take what's there, unformed,
and work it somehow,
feel it and work it
like clay in my hands
and make it appear
there
where I can see it.

It feels finished
for a little while.
And then the longing arises
again,
a different kind.
It requires the other
to listen,
to touch,
to hold.

But I can never write for you.
I can only write for me
and hope.

I think it is essential for each of us to find our own ways of creating sacred space, of moving inward and deepening, of accessing and honoring the language of soul.

My exploration reflects a more feminine structure to fit the feminine aspects of process and content of the soul journey. Women's work has traditionally been circular and piecemeal rather than linear and direct. Women have been weavers and quilt makers: from disjointed threads they have woven whole cloth and from discarded bits of cloth they have fashioned new creations. I have attempted to work the threads and scraps of my personal experience and the experiences of other women into a meaningful whole, and the process has been a spiraling journey reflecting the movement of psyche. Figures and images appear and reappear as meanings shift and deepen. I have circled around the central fact of cancer, enriching it with associations and amplifications. The spiral shape of the process, a series of circles of meaning reflected in this writing, is faithful to the spirit of the work and emphasizes that it is the journey rather than the destination which is essential.

Throughout the book I use dreamwork as one way of accessing and exploring unknown aspects of myself, and I use poetry as a way of speaking from my soul. In chapter 2, "A Vision of Soul," I present my understanding of a sense of soul as the foundation of this exploration and discuss the idea of "seeing through" reality to look at soul. The remaining chapters deal with circles of meaning and metaphor that have gathered around the lump of cancer for me. In chapter 3, "A View of Feminine Consciousness," I focus on the image of an empty box which contains the move into interiority and symbolizes feminine consciousness in its completion of emptiness. In chapter 4, "Symptom and Symbol," I discuss illness as metaphor, as an initiating call to transformation and as a pull to body and Self, and I describe my first encounter with an inner figure. In chapter 5, "Images of Self," I circle around the image of a tree as a symbol of the Self as it presented itself to me in active imagination. In chapter 6, "The Temple of Women," I share experiences of sand tray work and active imagination that honor a new vision of the feminine, and I explore the cancerous silence of women in our society. In chapter 7, "A Blaze for the Journey," I use the metaphor of a blaze cut into a tree and look at journeying beyond the limits of ego, contrasting the values of having and being. In chapter 8, "The Journey Continues," I look back on the process of creating this work and discuss fears and ongoing issues of time, space, and creativity. In "Final Thoughts," I reflect on the journey and on the lessons and questions that remain with me.

INTERLUDE

Speaking of Fairy Godmothers

There were thirteen of them in the kingdom,
thirteen fairy godmothers,
wise women or witches, as you wish,
but there were only twelve gold plates for the celebration.
You see the problem
already:
it is always with the uninvited guest,
the rejected aspect,
the disowned self.
Gold plates are so important, after all,
so shining and substantial.

So they each of them, the godmothers,
eleven of them in turn
gave blessings to the child,
gifts and powers and riches,
and she moved through the years,
half a lifetime and more.

And then the thirteenth spoke, out of turn.
When the thirteenth speaks
she always interrupts
where we think we are.
And there was darkness in the land.

But the twelfth had yet to be heard.
She appeared in black,
as she usually does,
skirts swirling streaks of gold,

not like the plates, though,
more like flashes of brilliant light and beckoning laughter.
She spoke softly but with sureness:
she knew all about curses and spells and antidotes
and the long forgotten art of making gold.

"It will not always be so," she said,
and quietly took her place in the circle
of women.
And it wasn't.

It's a long ago story
of gold plates and spells and falling asleep
and briars growing around
hiding, closing off, deadening.
We all sleep through it
most of the time,
and worry about the number of gold plates on the shelf,
and forget about the uninvited thirteenth
and the inevitable curse of darkness.

Until we don't.

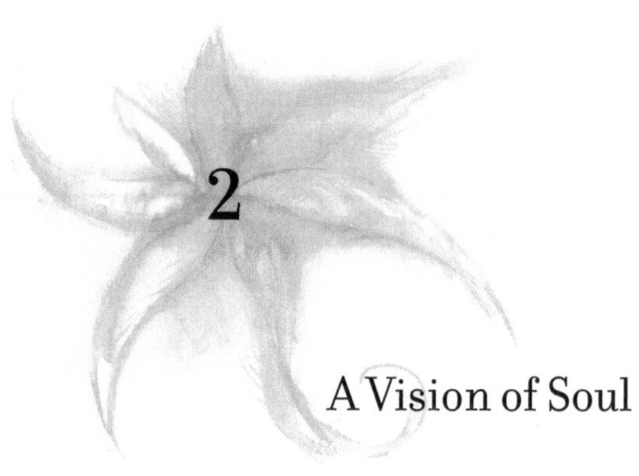

2

A Vision of Soul

And who will care, who will chide you if you wander away from wherever you are, to look for your soul?

—Mary Oliver, "Have You Ever Tried to Enter the Long Black Branches"

I HAVE LEARNED that the process of seeing metaphorically involves a movement away from the narrow viewpoint of ego, the more limited, mostly conscious aspect of oneself, and toward the larger viewpoint of the totality of psyche which encompasses both conscious and unconscious aspects. Ego likes to be in control and believes that it can be and that it is; psyche often challenges that stance.

Individuation, becoming more fully oneself, embraces the idea of wholeness rather than perfection; it includes a search for unconscious elements within oneself. A symptom, either psychological or physical, is not simply to be eradicated in the quest for perfection but can be explored for the meaning and wisdom it may carry.

To begin to explore an understanding of such a method of seeing, I recall a dream I had around the time of my cancer diagnosis. In the dream, I am taking the broken figures from my chess set to a shoe repairman to have them fixed. I am furious with him because he is the one who had broken them, and I want him to acknowledge the damage and repair them. The man in the dream is Gérard Depardieu, the French actor, who represents to me a man of earthiness, of body, of lusty appetites, of intense sensuality and sexuality.

It was hard to get beyond the rage I felt at this dream figure to see through to any value or wisdom, just as it is always difficult for the ego to let in the other. The ego experiences defeat and death when it is asked to incorporate a larger perspective; ego will fight to maintain a superior position and will resist the undermining efforts of psyche.

The chess pieces seem to suggest the intellectual aspects of ego, the pieces of a mind game. They were broken by a man who presents a more embodied aspect, perhaps the earthiness and vitality of libido. But I take the broken pieces to this man, the man who repairs soles/souls. Ego must be broken apart and then repaired or reassembled, much like the initiation of the shaman or the underworld journey of the hero. For a woman like me who feels safest in her head, the raw force of body and appetite may be experienced as a man, as the different other. Such a demand for change may feel similar to the abduction of the innocent Persephone by Hades in the Greek myth, a demand of the underworld forces, a pulling down into the earth, into body, into the depths. It is a destruction of innocence and a demand for expanded consciousness–in this case a kind of body consciousness. With cancer, I felt called to a deeper awareness of my body involving both a physical need to nurture it and a psychological need to explore it for meaning.

Since my illness, my root metaphor for a depth perspective has been the image of cancer. It is the lump that grew in my body, close to my heart, becoming the secret around which my soul grew. It is that experience which has called me most forcefully to the underworld, which has demanded a breaking up of the chess pieces of ego and a repairing of psyche, of soul. It is that which has called me to body.

I believe this is a crucial aspect of a Jungian orientation: to attend to and honor the centrality of psyche which is known and experienced as image. Such an approach involves a valuing of soul and a trusting of soul wisdom to heal itself and to journey toward wholeness. It attends to the longing of the soul in the symptom and believes in the primacy of the image and the power of the symbol to heal. It welcomes the plurality of psyche and honors the gods within the illness. It creates space for both silence and play, and it creates the vessel for containment and for the connection of relationship.

As I sought to make meaning of my cancer, I found myself drawn to honoring soul. Elusive and difficult to define, soul suggests to me a sense of deepening, of connecting with the essential aspect of oneself, of connecting with the Divine. The nature of soul contains the mystery of paradox. Soul both longs for the solitude of inner space and silence and is hungry for union with the soul of another, with the soul of creation, with the Divine. It is motionless and constantly moving: timeless, eternal, and always in the immediacy of the moment. As T. S. Eliot writes, "at the still point, there the dance is."[1]

If we are to attempt to approach soul, we may need to move as soul does, taking the indirect way, circling around. The step becomes a bit more tentative, the voice slightly hushed, the gaze softer. Soul speaks in whispers, in the breath of life and the movement of a breeze; soul speaks in image, in metaphor, in symbol. It can be as powerful as a symphony or an ocean, but when we touch soul we are somehow quieted, slowed. We approach the mystery with reverence. Soul seeks the meandering path rather than the straight line: as water moves always downward seeking the depth, so soul is in motion, seeking to go deeper.

To describe soul, I need to turn to the language of the poets, the language of image. I have long loved the words of Gerard Manley Hopkins: "there lives the dearest freshness deep down things."[2] Deep down aliveness, an intense and compelling vitality, begins to suggest what soul is. Gaston Bachelard speaks of the "values of inwardness" and says to meet soul, one must always "move closer."[3] Soul is deep down all things: one experiences soul deep down within oneself and within all creation, so that soul is inside and outside at once; as one moves closer, one experiences the intimacy of this connection. May Sarton writes of Ulysses who "shaped his course homeward at last toward the native source, seasoned and stretched to plant his dreaming deep."[4] It is this sense of coming home, of returning to the source, of planting and dreaming deep that speaks of soul to me.

I see the art of inner psychological work much like the art of poetry: both are in the service of honoring the image of soul. Both focus on the unique expression of the individual psyche to speak deeply of the nature of the reality of self and the world. I found descriptions in the worlds of poetry and psychology that capture the essence of this kind of vision and expression. Emerson said, "the poet turns the world to glass."[5] And Russell Lockhart echoes the metaphor when he states: "psyche, like poetry, turns reality into glass so that soul can be seen and heard."[6] It is the glass of soul that we look at and in to see the essential centering of soul.

I have on a table in my study a small glass box, empty: it is an image of the vision promising to put psyche at its center. The glass itself speaks of soul seeing, a kind of seeing into and through. The space within is the space of soul, the room to move and play, the innerness, the emptiness, the silence of depth. The box suggests the notion of container, of vessel, of that which holds the process and allows the time of waiting.

I experience soul as a longing for connection with the silence and space within myself, a reaching so deep within myself that I touch the God who is both within and not within, that I touch the depth of the soul of the world in which I live and which comes alive in me. Soul lives deep within me, and when I am in touch with it, I live more deeply in and into the world. It is, in Rainer Maria Rilke's sense of things, a "living into" the questions and answers of life, a living into the depths of one's own being and the being of the world.[7]

The territory of the soul is circular and spiraling, never linear and direct. I envision it as a series of circles without physical dimension, circles which suggest both deepening and opening at once. Some of my favorite poets have imagined such circles. Wallace Stevens touches such a mystery in the following lines from his poem, "Thirteen Ways of Looking at a Blackbird":

> When the blackbird flew out of sight,
> It marked the edge
> Of one of many circles.[8]

Such a series of circles, unseen, uncounted, seem to suggest the landscape of soul. These are invisible circles, perceptible only as the blackbird flies, edges marked only as they are experienced.

Rilke too writes of the unknowable circles of living soul:

> I live my life in growing orbits
> which move out over the things of the world.
> . . . .
> I am circling around God, around the ancient tower,
> and I have been circling for a thousand years,
> and I still don't know if I am a falcon, or a storm,
> or a great song.[9]

Such circles of soul seem to create depth and expansiveness at the same time, moving around the center, spiraling down and opening out in an invisible pattern of motion.

When we speak of soul, I think we must always turn to the

image, to the metaphor, to the symbol, because it is the essence of soul. It is there we must go to see through, mining under ego for the treasure. It is image that can best contain the plural and paradoxical nature of things. The power of the image is its ability to draw us in, move us closer, quiet us to hear the whispers of soul. It enchants us into paying attention and can carry us beyond our usual perspective. Bachelard tells us images are more compelling than ideas. They "seduce us through all our senses" and lead us inevitably to the world of metaphor.[10] The image of a glass box called to me long before I understood its significance.

Soul loves the freedom of movement, the loosening of the literal which can create inner spaciousness for soul play. This space allows room for the inner child to live, and room to connect with this child in play. Bachelard reminds us we must stay in contact with this place of childhood, of imagination, because it "remains a source of life deep within us, a life that stays in harmony with the possibilities of new beginnings."[11]

I believe the soul craves what we often think of as downtime. I have heard many women talk about feeling depleted by life's tasks. When they are able to connect with their inner longings for restorative healing, they often discover needs for having time alone, for connecting with nature and the Divine, for finding ways to express creativity. I have always felt such a pull; cancer has intensified the urgency.

Soul needs to be fed by creativity and a sense of time-out-of-time. I experience soul as the part of me that feels ageless, that hasn't changed over the years. I think it is similar to the part of me that gets lost in timelessness when I am engaged fully in creative expression of any kind. After a session of painting or writing or photography, it's as if I return to a present reality from a very different place. I look up from my palette or pencil or camera lens, and I am often surprised at how much time has passed.

When we do inner psychological work, we should, like the poet, always search for the image. The dream is often at the center of the work, for it is in the dream where images and symbols of the unconscious are most readily available. But there are other ways of accessing inner images: some I will explore are sand tray work, active imagination, drawing, and journaling.

What about the meaning of images and symbols in the work? Again, poetry and psychological work seem to share a goal of not rushing too quickly to interpretation. Archibald MacLeish wrote: "A poem should not mean / But be."[12] Symbols are not to be translated into other words but rather to be held in the fullness of their complexity. James Hillman speaks of the same danger in a psychological sense and cautions us against trying to reshape the images of psyche into something else. "We sin against the imagination whenever we ask an image for its meaning, requiring that images be translated into concepts."[13] In the honoring of psyche, one does not want to interpret the image into something else; the dream, like the poem, is its own best and richest communication. And yet we want to let meaning emerge, eventually, in its own time. The images need to be held loosely and respectfully, not tightly squeezed into some other shape or meaning. One must be careful to respect the symbol and explore its intricate layers of meaning with caution and care.

The journey of soul, through soul, is circular, spiraling deeper and wider in the paradoxical movement of psyche. It is the attempt to see through the glass of reality and to enter the space of play. It is to trust and honor the image and to believe in the healing potential of the symbol. It is to journey back home and to return to the source. It is to know the God within oneself and to know the Self anew.

Through image we see soul, reach soul. My work is an attempt to put cancer behind glass, into glass, to allow the process of soul-making to occur. It is to enter the world of the imaginal to explore there the psychic realities enriching and deepening the experience of illness. It is the journey of soul, to soul.

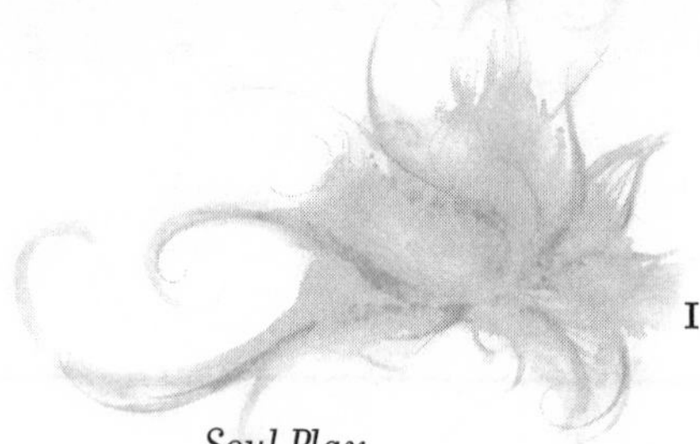

INTERLUDE

Soul Play

Chaos may grow
out of control
in the body
of one who wants to be
spirit.
It may scream inside
the one who yearns
too urgently
for silence.

Psyche doesn't like the seesaw at rest,
one end planted firmly in the dry dirt
of the abandoned playground,
the other pointed too high
toward the gods.

A seesaw is for playing:
soul loves to be in motion,
balanced for a moment
and then flying free again,
delighting in the craziness
of the ride.

Hermes may jump suddenly on one end,
startling the unsuspecting rider perched carefully opposite,
shaking him loose,
even throwing him off.
Hades may reach up to the elevated seat,
yanking it abruptly down,

down into his realm
of the depths.

One never knows who will enter the game
when psyche plays.
Chaos
may be exactly
what is needed.

3

A View of Feminine Consciousness

Once the soul awakens, the search begins and you can never go back.

—John O'Donohue, *Anam Cara*

I REMEMBER how I came to have the glass box. As I wandered through my inner landscape soon after the experience of cancer, I was drawn to an image of a box. Somehow, in ways I didn't yet understand, I knew it was a kind of treasure. I realized I wanted to find a box to embody this image, and I began to search for one that felt right. I looked at all kinds of containers: large and small, wooden, brass, and silver, plain and decorated. Gradually, I knew it had to be clear glass so that I could see the emptiness and feel the space inside.

I thought it might be like an unopened present, beautifully wrapped and ribboned and containing the possibility of almost anything. Opened, no matter how special, it could only be one thing. But unopened, it could be anything and everything; it was potentiality unlimited. It could contain the heart's desire before it was articulated or even known. It could be a favorite new book, a beautiful jewel, a piece of blue sky.

At first it seemed the box was possibility, potential, waiting to be actualized and empowered somehow, filled up. And yet that didn't feel right. The beauty of the box, the meaning of the box, seemed still to be in its emptiness. I loved to see and feel and enjoy the inner space of the box. It was peaceful and still and expansive, never confining or restricting. And it was more and more clearly the treasure itself.

An empty box, the treasure? What did it mean? I kept feeling the pull toward space both externally and internally. I sought out the writings of other women who treasured such times of solitude, and I savored their stories. As I was immersed in the ordinary details of life, I longed for a time of aloneness, of space and quiet and reflection, the emptiness of the box.

The inner images became more definite and more compelling: long walks by the ocean and home to a fire and some tea, lots of books, paper and pen, no schedule. Or time in a room, wrapped in a quilt and wrapped in thought, watching the weather outside, perhaps, but mostly watching the weather within me. Nobody else to do for. The chrysalis period, curled up around myself to let change happen.

There was a pull within toward more time for interiority, for contemplation and prayer and reflection. Time for poetry and music. Time to read without the strong light of focused energy, with permission to wander down any path that seemed intriguing. Time to dream. No appointments, no lists, no clocks. I remember the luxury of taking a whole day to rest and restore my energy.

> A perfect day:
> cold sleet on the streets
> built a moat of excuses
> to keep me in.
>
> All day in my old pink terry robe,
> most of the time in bed,

pillows piled behind my back in thick comfort.
I wrote
and I read
and I made a cappuccino with extra foam
just for me.
I luxuriated in the quiet
and the expanse of unscheduled time.

A kind of sick day,
it might appear,
but the healthiest one in months.

Just for me.

But it was more than rest I sought. I felt a deepening into myself to find the essence, still partly elusive somehow after all these years. And I felt a need to nourish the Self, the deeper and more inclusive part of me, to attend to its needs and wants. I longed for empty space and time to allow myself to be; I craved a feeling of inner spaciousness. And then I found words from James Hillman to help me to understand the meaning of my search. He describes such emptiness as "the lacuna of the feminine void," something which is "not to be overcome, fulfilled, completed." Rather, he says, "the emptiness is the completion, so that this lacuna becomes the place of reflection, the place of psychic awareness . . . it is psyche itself."[1]

"The emptiness is the completion." I felt the words resonate within me, and I knew the deep truth of which he spoke. I realized that this is the essential aspect of feminine consciousness and that it is crucial to honor this quality of emptiness. It is not a receptacle waiting to be filled with masculine energy of thrusting and doing. It must be cherished in its own right: the emptiness as completion, not lack.

As I wondered how to translate the meaning of this insight into living reality, I became aware that the image was changing. Slowly the box became larger, a whole room to walk around in, a house to live in. I began to understand it meant, first of all, not to leap too quickly to meaning, not to reduce but to enlarge, not to answer but to look for more questions, not to seek easy equivalents but to allow oneself to expand inside the metaphor.

It seems to encompass many feminine issues: the woman who needs a man to complete her life, the woman who needs to eat or drink or shop to fill the emptiness inside, the woman who feels she has been playing a series of roles all her life and has never discovered her essence, her Selfness deep within.

It may involve a process of clearing out the clutter, of going through the closets and drawers and refrigerator and cupboards and getting rid of what doesn't fit any more, what doesn't nourish any more: the old ways of being, the habits, the patterns of early family dynamics, the roles taken on to please others. Sometimes one has to work very hard just to get to the empty space.

It will involve destruction and certain deaths, this process of clearing away the old. It brings death to what has been outgrown, to what has become too easy and comfortable and safe. It often feels like death to let go and venture into the emptiness, sometimes dark and frightening. It is a death of ego to search for Self, the deeper and more complete aspect of one's being. And it is a time of birth.

I found myself drawn to the experiences of women who have made this kind of journey, who have learned that it involves a time of emptiness, space, solitude, death. It seems this is a need felt by many women, and I wanted to connect with their visions, their words. Alice Koller shares some of her process of clearing away during her winter in Nantucket, a season of solitary reflection and inner exploration. She describes how she has to let go of all her old habitual behaviors as she learns to choose ruthlessly exactly what she wants. And she lists for us the many ways in which we play false to self, the ways in which we settle for what doesn't fit or nourish or reflect who we are within.

> But think of all the ways there are to lie and I've done every one of them. Pretending to like something because someone in authority does. Evading a question. Saying only part of what I believe. Not saying anything at all. Shaping my words to fit what I know will be acceptable. Smiling when someone intends to be funny. Looking serious when my thoughts are elsewhere. Agreeing when I haven't even thought over the matter. Drawing someone out just because I know he wants to talk. Trying to amuse in order to avoid talking about something I'm not sure of.[2]

It's a list which may be familiar to many women, I suspect.

Kim Chernin has also spent a season of solitude in search of self. She speaks of a "longing to peel back layer after layer of pretense, compliance, and accommodation so that I could stand naked before myself as a woman."[3] She talks about the reinventing of herself, the time of in-between-ness that must be endured, when one must live with "The Woman Who Is Not Yet." I loved this image of a part of oneself that must be held, and honored, and waited for. It is for Chernin a time of "giving birth, the way women do, with mighty labor and a lot of blood."[4] It can be a time of pain and fear, and also a time of hope.

Marion Woodman writes of an inner voice calling to us, "whispering, 'It's not worth it. There's nobody here. I need a cocoon. I need to go back and find myself.'"[5] And she affirms the necessity of the process. "That is what going into the chrysalis is all about–undergoing a metamorphosis in order one day to be able to stand up and say *I am*."[6] Again there is a mixture of fear and hope.

Alix Shulman writes of the same kind of journey. She left behind a busy life to live for a while in a simple and solitary existence on an island off the coast of Maine in what she calls the "purity of silence."[7] She asks herself, "And what will send me soaring and plunging? I want to avoid contaminating the answer by imposing my will but simply watch patiently and see. I'm prepared to slow down, wait, even stop–whatever it takes to get a true reading."[8] She describes her transformation: "My ambitious ego-driven will, that muscular taskmaster I've cultivated for years and honored with obedience, ambles languidly in the sun, awaiting my orders. Instead of leading, it seems content to follow along wherever I want to go."[9] The inner bully has become an ally.

What of our own individual journeys, our own inner experiences of the treasure, the psyche? I think of the Greek goddess Artemis as the guide for this kind of soul journey, for it is she who can pull us away from the world and into the secret, silent places. She has several attributes that can help us in our inner wanderings and searching. She is the goddess of the hunt and of the wilderness, so she can companion us on our inner exploration of wilderness and hunt for connection to soul. She is the goddess of childbirth, so she can help midwife the birth of a newly emerging authenticity. And she is a virgin goddess in the sense of psychological virginity, strong in her sense of self and inner conviction.

And so I return to the emptiness of the box. It is there we must journey to find depth, to find meaning, to find soul. It is to live in the fullness of emptiness that gives space for the metaphor to emerge, for the Self to unfold. It is never an easy task. But we must learn to tolerate stillness and silence if we are to connect with our own souls, to allow the metaphor to be and not need it to mean too quickly, to allow the chrysalis to endure as long as it takes, to allow the death of the old before the birth of the new. From the image of the box, we can remember the importance of holding and containing, to host and honor the psyche. It can be the vessel in which transformation occurs, in which birth happens. It teaches the way of being with dreams, to question and explore and expand and to allow the symbol to transform. It is itself the metaphor in which to live.

It may not require a season alone by the ocean or in a room of one's own, but it does involve following Artemis away from the world to the hidden paths, the unknown and undiscovered places. It is a time of dying to the old and giving birth to the new and enduring the pain of the process. It is a time of solitude and stillness, of going deep within the self to the silent space, to find the emptiness that is the completion, the treasure.

INTERLUDE

The Seduction of Order

I want my world to be a Zen garden.
I rake the sand carefully
each morning
and place the stones
just so
in some illusion of beauty
and meaning.

And then I look away
and something is thrown in from just beyond the edges:
it splatters in the sand
and destroys the pattern.
At night
things grow from below:
they burst through
at will
crowding out the order
and the attempt at peace.

Truth
is so messy
and inconvenient.
And is the point of the garden
after all
to organize
or to ensoul?

4

Symptom and Symbol

In dreams we go down, as if pushed down into our depths by the hands of God. Pushed down and planted in our own inner land, the roots suck, the bulb swells. In her depths everything grows in silence . . .

—Meinrad Craighead, *The Litany of the Great River*

A PHYSICAL SYMPTOM, like a psychological symptom, may point the way to a desire of psyche. It may be an embodiment of the "dis-ease" existing in the whole person, the totality of body-mind-psyche. Such a symptom may occur when there is a lack of harmony throughout the system because energy is not flowing freely. I am not so much interested in attempting to look at linear causality but rather to circle around the issue: both in larger circles, around the metaphor of illness as expressive of needs of the psyche, and in smaller circles, around the particular metaphorical meanings that connect with breast cancer for me.

Body workers and practitioners who work with the energy of the body understand the interconnectedness of body, mind, spirit, and soul. There are many modalities that address these links: therapeutic touch, healing touch, acupuncture, Reiki, and shamanic healing are some examples. From them we learn that emotions and experiences are somehow stored in the physical body, and we unconsciously tighten parts of the body in response to something perceived as a threat, either physical or emotional. As a physical example, many people have experienced a tightening of back muscles that constrict in a painful attempt to prevent further injury. Something similar happens with feelings; somehow we constrict parts of ourselves to try to protect against further pain. Practitioners who work with energy can often sense these blockages where energy doesn't flow freely.

I wanted to learn more about the mind-body connection so I began to work with a practitioner of Hakomi, a body-centered therapy that involves paying attention to physical sensations, images, feelings, memories. As I entered a contemplative state, I had an immediate and powerful image-experience of an old reality in my body. My felt experience was of a curved bar of iron pressed against my chest, pushed into my chest. I saw and felt and understood that this was an old issue; I had tightened and contracted and almost curled myself around this external force so that my shoulders hunched in a kind of protective, armored stance. It felt like a cringe of fear, a memory and an expectation and a defense against attack. It was an extremely strong and surprising image, and I felt some of its grip dissolving with my tears of compassion for myself. Reflecting later on the experience, I was, of course, struck by the location of the image in the area of my cancer. The mystery of body-knowing continues to haunt me.

Psyche can speak through illness in various ways. Illness intensifies the experience of life: it raises the ante by making the reality of death much more immediate. One knows in a new and powerful way that life is not forever, and one knows how crucial it is to live life fully, and fully as oneself.

There are many ways in which this can occur, but the image of cancer seems to be especially apt. Cancer cells can perform only the function of growth; they are primitive cells, threatening to the organism because they grow out of control, consuming. Cancer is an image of energy gone awry, of growth perhaps demanded by the psyche but not enacted by the person. Such powerful energy for growth will not be denied; thwarted, it twists itself into a negative and destructive form.

Illness is an initiation, a call to consciousness, and a summons to transformation. It is a tearing away of the old and a forceful pull into the underworld of loss and death. It is a path never chosen, but one that may be embraced as a way of individuation. By stripping away the masks of persona and undermining the usual props and defenses of ego, illness forces a movement away from self-image and into a more authentic self.

More specifically, illness pulls one directly and dramatically into the body, forcing one "to care for oneself at the most elemental level," says Judith Duerk, "that of matter itself." In illness, she says, "finally, comes permission to rest, permission to treat with love and kindness the base matter of one's own body."[1] In cancer, attention is drawn powerfully to this cellular level; one becomes aware of the cells in one's body and focuses attention and consciousness there in a new way.

Illness has gotten my attention: it has left me naked before the mirror of reality. It needs to be listened to much as we listen to dreams. Both speak to us through metaphor, through the power of the image, through the circular and meandering route rather than the fast and linear one. It is about meaning, not cause, which can give us the link between the fact of illness and the meaning of illness; it can transform diagnosis into image.

Malignancy: the word is very difficult to hear as a diagnosis. When the surgeon called that February evening, his voice was calm as he gave me the details of the options available to me: mastectomy or lumpectomy with chemotherapy and radiation. I know I tried hard to take in all he was saying, even as part of me was thinking this couldn't be right, there must be a mistake, the test results must have gotten mixed up. I moved through the next few days in a numb fog of deadened feeling, probably necessary for the decision-making process to occur. I had to weigh the pros and cons of various methods and strategies and cut through the medical opinions and research with a blade as sharp as the surgeon's would have to be. Eventually I underwent a lumpectomy, followed by the suggested chemotherapy and radiation.

I experienced the loss of persona that illness brings, first in the disfigurement of my breast and then, strangely even more intensively, in the loss of my hair during chemotherapy. A deformed breast calls for private tears, a solitary woman staring in the bathroom mirror, trying to come to terms with the mutilation of her body, or with her lover, struggling to retain her feelings of sexuality in a changed body. This is by far the deeper pain. But the loss of hair is such a public humiliation, so apparent for all to see. Even hidden under a wig, I felt such a longing to be normal again, just to be ordinary.

I remember when I went shopping for a wig. Because I elected to have an aggressive form of chemotherapy, I knew I would lose my hair very soon into the treatment. A good friend came with me to help me deal with the emotional challenges. I tried on many different looks, almost as one would try on hats to see the different effects. Some were similar to my own hair and some were quite different, like playing with different personalities. We laughed at some of the more outrageous possibilities, but in the end I stayed with a choice that was similar to my own hair. Looking back, it was probably, at least in part, an attempt to appear to be the same as I was before cancer, both to myself and to others.

The loss of hair symbolized and concretized the loss of persona that occurs with illness. It pulled me out of the ordinary world and forced me to live in the world of cancer. Every morning when I woke up I had to face my new image. My husband lovingly called me "Iggle," for bald eagle, and we could joke about it sometimes. But it was hard. Even as I gave thanks daily for being alive and for hopefully being free of cancer, I mourned the loss of an aspect of myself that was difficult to let go of. Stripped of persona props of normalcy and attractiveness, I felt ugly, different, alienated. When I appeared for the first time in public without my wig, my hair was very, very short. I deliberately allowed myself to feel a little naked and vulnerable, and I also realized I felt more free.

I found some comfort in an article by Alice Walker about a spiritual dilemma involving her relationship with her hair. She described feeling the experience of growth to be like a seed needing to push through the earth to become a plant, but she was distressed to find she "seemed to have reached a ceiling in [her] brain." She finally identified what she felt to be the "last barrier to spiritual liberation": her relationship to her hair.[2] After years of spending a lot of time thinking about her hair, she said she understood finally why nuns and monks shaved their heads. She felt she had "broken through the seed skin" and began to experiment with letting her hair display its own willfulness "to grow, to be itself . . . to be left alone."[3]

I too struggled with the lessons of my hair, both when I lost it and when it began to grow back in twisted waves that had not been there before. I thought about issues of letting go and letting be, of moving away from the safety of persona into a more authentic and vulnerable self. I never welcomed the teachings, but I tried to attend to them in spite of my discomfort.

The symptom of cancer and the symbol of cancer: I begin to walk around the images. The symptom of cancer is growth out of control; perhaps the symbol of cancer is a call to growth for the individual. The language of symptoms, body wisdom, is like dream language; an image is not the same for all dreamers and must be understood in context, in the particular story of the individual. But there may be archetypal images, universal themes transcending the specific meanings.

Cancer cells are primitive cells, reflective of primitive, early feelings and needs pushing for growth. I think of bulbs planted in a shiny green ceramic bowl in my kitchen, placed there to bring color and life to the midwestern winter that can be too long and too gray. I see how tender the young shoots seem to be when they first appear, delicate and fragile wisps of green, but how forcefully they thrust their way through even the thickest clumps of earth, seeking the sun and their own flowering. They require a time of darkness in the earth so that nutrients can be absorbed and transformation can occur.

So all growth pushes for actualization; all energy yearns for fulfillment. Growth of cancer cells in a time of darkness may be related to growth of the person, requiring a time of rest, a connection with the nurturing earth. I met my cancer with imagery of green for healing: an attempt to heal growth with growth, like curing like.

Green
for healing:
expanse of lawn,
smooth and restful;
leaves
uncurling
and opening upward
toward the sun;
slender shoots
pushing through the earth
to be born
and bloom.

Life emerges again every spring;
it's one of the things I love most
about
winter.

So with cancer,
green
for healing.

Emerald power
pulling in light and energy.
Sunshine
and prayer
and green for healing.

As I continued to explore meanings connected to my breast cancer, I came to realize there was a link to the image of mother: to my actual mother; to the mother figure within myself, capable of nurturing me and others; to the mother I have been to my children; and to the archetypal mother figure in various forms.

It began with a dream. I started keeping a dream journal when I was forty years old, and the first dream I recorded was one in which my mother had given me cancer because she hadn't fed me properly when I was an infant. Seven years later, the cancer appeared, and the images of cancer and mothering and feeding began to intertwine. I thought of my mother, who hadn't nursed me, whose milk didn't flow from her breasts, whose ability to nurture was not easy and free. And I thought of myself as a mother, also choosing not to nurse my children, taking in attitudes from my mother as totally as I would have taken her milk. Not getting enough? Not giving enough? My questions are not about the literal issue of breast feeding rather than bottle feeding, although it may play a part. Rather they circle around the issues that are symbolized by the breast, by the nurturing and feeding capacities of the breast.

I want to be careful to explore meaning rather than cause, but I find myself wondering about a psychological link between mother and daughter in the disease of breast cancer. The hereditary factor for breast cancer between mother and daughter is acknowledged to be very strong. Perhaps attitudes about mothering and nurturing, feeding and eating, trusting and fearing, giving and receiving can all be passed from mother to daughter as powerfully as genetic components. As a mother feeds her daughter, so she feeds herself, so her daughter learns to feed herself and others. A mother passes on her beliefs and attitudes about how to be a wife, a lover, a mother, a daughter–how to be a woman.

I remember trying to look more deeply into the meaning by writing about the lump in my breast:

> I have a rock
> near my heart
> where it should be mother soft and flowing.
>
> I have tried to soften it
> with tears,
> but it remains.
>
> A small rock,
> a stone perhaps,
> not even noticeable
> outside,
> but rock hard
> solid fury
> and pain.

The fury surprised me. I knew of personal pain, but I was not in touch with the level of rage present in this hard place. It wasn't until later that I made a connection between my anger and the cultural silencing of women.

The image of the breast is itself circular; I move around and around it in circles and let the images appear. The breast: supposed to be soft, womanly, feminine, sexy, nurturing, feeding, giving, yielding. Milk given or not given, withheld, blocked.

The image of a lump in the breast. A rock. A stone. A part of myself has turned into stone. Inside, deep inside the flesh it lies, not apparent to anyone outside, hidden, hard to detect. Hard, tight, a knot, a block, a twisted part. Lethal. Close to my heart it lies, life constricting and life threatening. Dammed up energy, snagged, cramped. A stuck place, tightened, tangled, snarled. It is an image of growth, uncontrolled: growth and control in a juxtaposition of opposites. In what ways have I felt out of control, do I feel out of control? I know a sense of drivenness and perfectionism that destroys the flow of being in the moment, of resting in and honoring the presentness of life. I recognize a knot of tightness and feel a need to let go of the convention and form of appropriateness and to rejoice in and be thankful for growth of authenticity.

I remember my first experience with active imagination, a Jungian technique used to connect with images and figures from the unconscious. Jung described it as "dreaming with open eyes."[4] I quieted my mind and focused on my inner world, inviting in any image that might want to come. I let myself imagine my cancer as something in psyche which wanted to speak to me; I wondered what it might be saying, what it wanted to teach me, what were its questions, its lessons, its gifts. I let myself imagine my cancer as an inner teacher and waited to see who or what might emerge.

A woman appears, tall, slender and cool, wearing long robes, gray-blue and flowing. She seems distant, perhaps alien, but not menacing. I have come to think of her as Soul Woman, the lady of the cancer, waiting, waiting to be born. She speaks to me of guilt and old pain and borrowed values, of the shell of the body and the invisible treasure, of death and rebirth and new meanings. She comes to remind me, to have me remember: that life is not forever, that there are limitations as well as myriad possibilities, that life is unbearably sweet and deeply painful, that there are endings and beginnings and often they are the same, that the answers are not as important as the questions.

She teaches me also in silence, about silence, about waiting in stillness. She reminds me of the lines from T. S. Eliot: to be still, to wait, "so the darkness shall be the light, and the stillness the dancing."[5] And so I learn, or try to learn, the lessons of wordlessness, of emptiness that is full in its completion, of life that is enriched because of death.

Soul Woman, summoned by cancer, speaks often without words. She has been a healing image, a balance to the external busyness of things and tasks. The growth she asks is inner, slow, almost imperceptible, but essential. It is not the rampant uncontrolled growth of cancer, nor is it the tightly knotted, fearful defense against growth. Her robes are flowing and loose, and she moves freely in them, an image of energy moving easily and without constriction.

Interesting that she is cool, at a time when cancer and chemotherapy and even menopause have served literally and metaphorically to heat things up, like a fire which cooks and transforms. She is the opposite of drivenness and perfectionism. Interesting, too, that she is so tall and straight. I might have expected, and even preferred, a bent and withered old crone, a more visible carrier of wisdom. Perhaps she has something to tell me about a part of myself still clinging to the straightness of convention and the comfort of rule. Or perhaps she has something to tell me about the need to stand up taller and straighter in my own life.

She teaches me about loosening the boundaries and walking out of prisons I have been carrying with me. She teaches me about letting go, of learning to die the little deaths along the way to prepare for the final death. She teaches me about breaking out of rule-boundedness and of creating spirit, of giving and receiving in honesty and trust. She teaches me about feminine simplicity which is the fruit of a universe of plenty, not of scarcity.

She reminds me of Mary, the mother of Jesus: robes of blue, a message of simplicity, an image of woman waiting, holding herself ready. An acceptance of God's will: a path, though not chosen, embraced. And she reminds me of Mary, sister of Martha, not concerned with tasks and accomplishments, sitting at the feet of Christ to listen and be in relationship.

She leads me to appreciate relationships with women even more than before. I feel a kinship with women who have had breast cancer, both the individuals I know and all the unknown women who are part of this sisterhood. And I value the friends who are important to me: the friends who share a history, the friends who like to discuss books and ideas, the friends who talk of their joys and sorrows and listen to mine, the friends who speak the truth. These are the conversations worth having; the superficiality of conventional socializing has no appeal.

She has taught me about the Great Mother archetype, the universal image of mother, clamoring for attention and demanding recognition. I have learned that if I do not accept and honor her in my life, in the matter of my body, she may become destructive. But she has also taught me that the mother archetype is not always destructive and consuming. I have a fear of others wanting too much from me, too much of me. I have known how to set boundaries, but perhaps sometimes tighter than necessary. I have known how to be a container for others, but sometimes at the expense of my own desires and needs. Now I am learning to be more conscious of boundaries and to set them differently, sometimes more loosely and sometimes more firmly. I have learned to be a container with more choice and discernment, for myself and for others.

Cancer has taught me much, and I continue to learn. It has been a gift, one which I did not choose but for which I am grateful. It is the dis-ease we experience pulling us toward our growing edges. Disease pulls us into ourselves, pulls us away from persona concerns and ego defenses and into the center of our being, the Self. Never a gentle invitation, it can wrench us out of our comfortable world as forcefully as Hades's abduction of Persephone. As with Persephone, illness can offer a loss of innocence and a call to consciousness.

Cancer has pulled me into the matter of my body, to the wisdom of cell energy. I continue to struggle with its lessons and its demands, and I continue to circle the metaphor of meaning. The question remains: What is the unconscious demanding? I continue to walk slowly, around and around, waiting, learning to love the inner spaciousness, the stillness which is the dancing.

INTERLUDE

The Cancer of Silence

There are two kinds of silence
I have learned about.

In one,
an old one,
a woman stands deadly still,
a bar of iron pressed across her chest,
pressed into her flesh
and the flesh grown over it
long ago,
and the body grown around it,
curled imperceptibly
in an almost invisible cringe.

There is another kind of silence,
much newer and without form,
the silence of remembering,
of knowing without words,
of drawing deep into the body of self
to trust there for the first time,
to stop the busyness,
to stop.
It is the silence of the earth
embraced.

Is it the fear
or the memory
of the hot iron bar branding into her flesh
that keeps her moving?

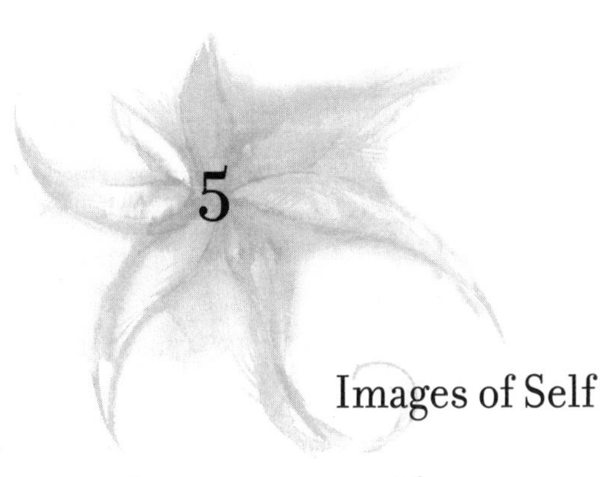

5

Images of Self

Once more, my cancer, I face you;
breathlessly, to fight and write
and furiously build; amassing blocks of
words against the shifting seasons . . .

—Whitney Scott, "Women Against the Shifting Season"

MY IMAGES OF CANCER continue to enlarge and grow, much like the cancer itself, but slowly, soulfully. Much like cellular growth, imaginal growth is irregular in shape and time—bumping out a little edge here, nudging a boundary there. The lines are not straight. Time and growth and causality are not linear: patterns are circular, cylindrical, cyclical. Images of Self appear, flow from one to another, connect and intertwine. I walk around and through them to learn the language and lessons of soul.

I think of my cancer as an image of the Self, a Jungian concept including both conscious and unconscious elements of psyche, both center and whole. A small, tight knot of hardness, the location of cancer is concretely anchored in one place in my body. But it becomes, for a time, the totality of my perception of my body. It threatens the whole body; it defines who I am on its own terms. It is not just my breast that had cancer—I had cancer.

A symbol of Self can be healing, in itself, and it can also carry wisdom and meaning that can assist on the journey toward wholeness. I spent some time one day entering a meditative state and seeking an image of Self; what appeared to me was a tree. A not uncommon image of Self, a tree represents natural growth unfolding at its own rate and in its own way. Beginning as a seed, it emerges slowly and fully into treeness. The image of a tree suggests groundedness in the earth and a reaching upward toward the sky and the sun. It is a study in connectedness and relatedness as it takes nutrients from the soil and the air and nourishes itself to provide health and growth.

I later explored some of the many archetypal associations and images connected with the tree to further understand layers of meaning in the symbol which had come to me. It is the tree of life and the tree of knowledge of good and evil in the garden of Eden. It is the shaman's tree, the axis connecting the underworld, middle world, and upper world. It is phallic masculine power and feminine cyclical regeneration. It is the Christian symbol of original sin and the redemptive power of the cross. It suggests cosmic life, immortality, fertility, the process of individuation.

My own imaginings of tree were haunted by a dream I had about a year earlier. In the dream, I am outside, near a house belonging to my parents. I am with my mother and father and two little girls who are also their daughters. I feel younger than my actual age. My mother and father have built an addition onto their house, up high and on the left side. It is an extra room, not designated for anything special, and can be reached by a new circular staircase on the outside of the room. I am very upset and sad because a large old tree has been killed in the process of building. At first, Mom and Dad say the tree will be fine, but I see they built the staircase too close to the roots; then I see the trunk was actually severed.

The scene changes then, and we are all inside, sitting together, as if for dinner. The youngest girl is on my lap. She is upset and tearful and says something about my father being abusive to my mother. I hold her as she cries and feel somewhat apart from the family as I tell them how concerned I am about the damage to the tree. My mother says something about catalogs and buying things and my father says it is nice to play tennis; I am distressed and tell him these answers have nothing to do with the tree.

I carried the dream with me for a long time and revisited and revisioned it often. It frightened me and appealed to me at the same time. I was terrified that the roots of the tree had been damaged and the trunk actually severed in two. I saw there were green leaves on the branches, but I knew, too, a tree could look healthy on the outside for a while but be damaged and dying inside.

Was this image of a tree about my body, or my soul, or both? I didn't know which I would prefer, which damage would be more bearable. I wondered about possible damage to my psyche, and I worried about a connection with my physical symptoms. I feared cancer may have been secretly growing again in my body, even while the outside looked healthy. I feared cancerous growth may have been secretly growing in my psyche, even while the outside looked strong.

I decided to make a drawing of the tree to see what might emerge on the page. Sometimes drawing an image from a dream or a meditation allows details to appear that are beyond our conscious awareness. I was surprised to see things I hadn't known before. The tree looked like a large old shade tree, probably a maple or an oak, with green leaves. The trunk was cut in two, and there was an actual gap of space between the two pieces, though the tree still stood. I felt echoes of my early images connected to cancer: the slash through the center of Georgia O'Keeffe's painting that created space and tension, and the gap which Annie

Dillard writes about that allows an opening for something larger to pierce our lives.

I could not see the roots of the tree to assess damage, but they were somehow able to hold the tree upright. What I hadn't seen until I drew the tree was that the trunk had grown, for a part of its life, almost directly sideways. It emerged from the ground straight up and then bent almost horizontal to the earth and grew to the left for a while before bending again and continuing its growth upward. Although I felt somewhat concerned about this irregular growth pattern, I also recognized an almost nostalgic feeling for the sideways part, as if I used to like to sit there and daydream, perhaps, or read and muse a little. Sideways felt less direct, less thrusting, a time of staying close to the earth, a sense of resting and of consolidation. As I thought about it later, it seemed it might have also signaled a kind of self-protection: Were there times in my life when I felt I had to keep myself safe by being less direct and forceful?

When I imagined the roots of the tree underground, they felt like my hands grasping very tightly, trying to hold firmly to the earth. It was as if I had to anchor the tree very strongly so it wouldn't be blown over by strong winds or fall because of its own unbalanced weight.

The killing of the tree in the dream frightened me when I concretized it and became worried about my own possible death from cancer. Gradually I began to accept the possibility that it was not necessarily a literal death that was imaged or called for, but a symbolic death of some part of me, some part of me that was damaged and split by my parents' building.

It was the circular staircase, built too close, that damaged the roots of the tree: a circular staircase, built of metal, mostly open. The circularity reminded me of growth, circular and cyclical. It seemed to be a feminine image, the circle of the breast itself, the circle of thinking which is meandering and gentle rather than linear and harsh. It connected to the circular rings of growth in the tree trunk, hidden from view but marking the pattern of years. And it seemed to be a masculine image, too: a product made of iron or steel, hardened to carry traffic, a connector between two levels, but not a natural organic one of reciprocity and relationship. A circular staircase seemed to belong inside but was placed outside in this dream, somewhat awkwardly and out of place.

The tree was an image of Self, both body and psyche: a feminine image of nurturing and growth, of renewal and regeneration. I realized I was afraid to trust the natural growth of treeness as it bends and turns. I wondered about the building of a staircase to move upward, a staircase which, though circular, is hard and unyielding. It seemed to be "outsiding" something which should be inner, which should be secret.

The secret was another image of Self: the center, the hidden, the unknown. I thought of Robert Frost's lines of poetry, "We dance round in a ring and suppose / But the Secret sits in the middle and knows."[1] Again I felt the presence of the theme of center and circumference, of center and wholeness, and I thought of cancer as a secret, hidden inside, unknown, imperceptible. As with the rings of growth in a tree, it cannot be detected from the outside and can only be seen when the knife cuts into the flesh, into the secret.

The tight knot of my cancer was like the knot of a tree, a place where the energy of life force gets twisted or blocked. Tree knots are outside and visible; cancer knots are inside and secret. The secret and the circle entwined: circular staircase, circular rings of life in a tree, circular breast. I felt called to dance around the circle to suppose, to begin to know. The secret Self within felt hidden and protected, not to be outsided too soon. The secret of the dream lived hidden inside, too.

I let my images meander, connecting loosely, flowing from one to another in tracings that were not linear. I thought of a large seashell, a nautilus, cut open to reveal a spiral pattern, like a staircase, like a tree, like a breast cut open to reveal its secret. It reminded me of part of the inner ear, an ear opened to hear the secret, to hear soulfully.

The shell has chambers, like so many different rooms in a house, like parts of Self. In the dream, there was a new room, an extra room, that was being added. I wondered if the dream was speaking of too much growth, cancerous growth, more than was needed? Too much growth, too close to the roots, damaging to the roots, cutting right through the trunk of the tree. I wondered about what kind of growth is healthy and what kind of growth is damaging. Cancer seems to offer teachings both about growth out of control and about growth rigidly resisted.

The damaged tree of the dream speaks of the lesson of growth that is abusive to the feminine and harmful to roots and trunk. In the dream, it is the masculine who is abusive to the feminine, though both ignore the reality of what is hurt and sad and dying. I felt myself to be both a daughter of my dream parents and separate from them. I was able to hold and comfort the smallest child within me, and I felt upset and sad, as she did, as we grieved the loss and pain of what is missing, what is damaged. I was both a part of the scene and apart from it: I seemed to be younger in the dream as I was pulled back into my childhood family, but I also know there are other rooms in my Self and that I, too, can build a new room when I need it.

I continue to dance around the secret of the tree and suppose. The root damage seems older, the trunk problem more recent. Both are damaged from the staircase, too close: the circular stairs feel too small, too confining. The circle should not be drawn too small, too tight. Sometimes the rings of growth of a tree are small, showing too little nourishment that year. Have I had times when I didn't have enough sustenance, enough nurturing? Have I failed at times to nourish myself? Circles which are drawn too small may shut out, exclude. Have I felt I've had to give outside access to my inner self when I didn't want to?

The room in my dream reminded me of my study, an important room for me; I think of it as a concretization of Virginia Woolf's "room of one's own" which provides the necessary solitude and privacy for a woman to be creative. My study is an upper room at the left side of the house. It is comfortable, with a soft chair and a warm blanket to wrap myself in. It holds some of my most special treasures: pictures of my family, favorite books, a seashell, a flowering plant, a small figure of a woman embodying the feminine to me, the glass box reminding me of the value and wisdom of emptiness. And it is waiting for other treasures: pieces of art I hope to find which are both beautiful and meaningful to me, perhaps one of an image of "my" tree.

The room itself is an image of Self, my most personal space. With a desk and bookcases and file cabinets, it is a place to work and study, to sort and order and contain. But it is also a place to read and write poetry and listen to music and meditate and dream. It has drawers with locks on them to contain the secrets that are important to keep safe. An upper room, it is reminiscent of the upper room of biblical reference, a place where the disciples waited for Jesus. It too can be a place of waiting for Self, of preparing with ego and waiting for grace. It can be a place of allowing growth and a place of luring growth.

The room in the dream was not mine, but a part of my parents' home. It did not honor the secret of Self but had an outside staircase to give access. It was empty, unfinished, unfurnished, extra. It did not have special treasures and keys and containers.

I continue to dance around my image of a tree, as the colored ribbons of the maypole twine and intertwine and weave a complex pattern. As there are many chambers in the nautilus shell, so there are many meanings in my dream. I look at the severed trunk in new ways. It may be about the need to cut into the cancerous breast to separate the good tissue from the diseased tissue. It may be about separations within the Self, between head and body, between mind and heart, between what is shown and what is hidden. It may also be about a positive need to sever part of the trunk, a need to separate from the roots of my parents in order to put down my own roots, a need to separate from the addition to my parents' house in order to more fully inhabit my own room.

As the tree is a symbol of nourishment and nurturance, so the dream image turned to one of dinner. But it is significant that in the dream we are merely sitting together as if for dinner; there is no food present. There is only the appearance of a setting for dinner, but not the actual feeding: form, but not substance. As I mourn the loss of the tree, and the young girl cries over the abuse of feminine by masculine, none of us are being fed. My mother speaks of shopping, and my father speaks of tennis; they do not even recognize the reality and pain of the violence nor do they care about the tree or the sadness of their daughters. They rush to fill the emptiness with things to buy and games to play.

In this dream, I am revisiting and healing old abuse of the feminine. There is a part of me that can grieve over the damage to the tree and can hold the child who needs to cry. But there may also be parts of myself that do violence to the young feminine within, that stay in irrelevant busyness to avoid the pain of loss.

I think of the tree outside our bedroom window. It is a large old maple reaching well above the second story of the house. When I went through chemotherapy for cancer I spent more time than usual in the bedroom, and I watched the tree change through the seasons. My treatments began in February when the branches were bare and etched a stark silhouette against the gray winter sky. Then spring began, and the green of new life started to appear: at first, the smallest traces, still more brown than green, as the earliest growth began to open. Then, day by day, more green unfurled until leafiness was fully born. In summer, it was wonderful to watch the dappled sunlight dance through the branches and enjoy the play of brightness and shadow against the green. Birds came to perch on its limbs and sing their melodies, and squirrels scampered, chattering loudly, leaping from one branch to another.

I noticed later, with some concern, that it had a peculiar kind of growth on some of its branches. When we consulted an expert to evaluate the problem and provide extra feeding for the tree, he said there was a fungus growing on it. Because of the severe drought the preceding summer, the tree had not gotten enough nutrients and was therefore more susceptible to disease. It may also have been affected by recent renovations to the house: walkways had been changed and landscaping had been redone, all close to the roots of this tree.

Like the tree of my dream, this tree may have sustained invisible damage to the roots. Like cancer, the fungus was able to take hold when the nourishment had been insufficient and the organism was weakened. Earlier, I had felt a connection with this tree and feared the loss of it, a portent of my own cancer and specter of death. But now I feel a new connection, more understanding and less fatalistic: if the tree dies, I will acknowledge and mourn the loss with pain, but I will also begin to understand that life includes death and is, in a way, completed by death. There is a force for decay as well as growth in all living things; that, too, is included in the image of Self.

I think of Georgia O'Keeffe's wonderful painting of a tree called *The Lawrence Tree.* To paint it from the perspective she wanted, she had to lie down on a bench under the tree and look up into the branches reaching into the sky. Her work turns our perspective upside down, and I think this is what is needed to understand the tree and the dream and cancer and Self.

The branches of O'Keeffe's tree, seen from underneath, look like roots. It is in seeing the underside of the tree that we seem to be seeing the under-side of the tree. As the branches twist out and disappear into the blackness of leafiness against a blue sky filled with stars, they look like roots reaching deep into the dark earth. Branches and roots alike speak of the paradox of separateness and similarity. O'Keeffe's image turns things upside down, or perhaps it turns us upside down. It cannot be understood in the usual way but must be approached from a turned-around upside-down place. It teaches us that we must turn ourselves in circles, like the playful cartwheeling of children, to approach the dream and the symbol and the Self.

I had another meditation session that day to revisit the image of Self, and I was surprised and even somewhat frightened by what I experienced. The tree of my dream appeared in my imagination, and slowly the trunk straightened itself out. The split slowly knitted itself together and healed, and the roots gently relaxed their overly tight grip on the earth. Even as I watched the changes occur, I had difficulty letting go of my tight grip on the old image. As I was afraid of the original symbol of the tree, so I was now afraid I was simply making this happen, that it was a manipulation to avoid the pain, that it was perhaps too simplistic and easy.

Gradually I was able to understand the message of growth of the tree, the organic growth that is not static and caught in one image, frozen and dead. I realized that it is about growth that sometimes bends when you think it should be straight and sometimes straightens when you think it should be bent. It is about healing occurring spontaneously and after a long time of preparation. And it is about roots holding the tree more firmly in the earth when they hold it loosely. The tree has become a significant image of Self to me, holding possibilities for new understandings and growth.

INTERLUDE

The Web

The web
of connectedness,
random,
but patterned,
contained.
Circular,
like the rings in a tree
marking growth,
like a staircase
too close to the roots
of an old tree.

The lifelines
woven fine:
a delicate structure,
but strong enough
to support.

A quietness of things,
hard stone
in a circle
almost,
and soft shells
whorled
and ancient.

Timeless and still
in the frame
of meaning,
ephemeral in form,
forever
in soul.

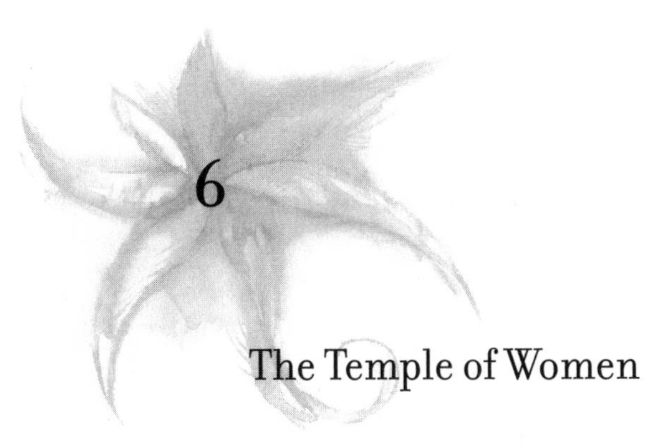

6

The Temple of Women

. . . a silence in which
another voice may speak.

—Mary Oliver, "Praying"

I CONTINUE TO WORK with images of cancer as I try to learn to let the disease heal my life. I am drawn within, not to my usual known place of safety in my head, thinking and analyzing, but to another, older, less familiar place. It is perhaps more like the sideways growth of the tree branch from my dream, closer to the earth, less direct and thrusting, more restful and timeless.

I return to explore the technique of active imagination, to delve into the meanings of cancer and the summons of psyche through the embodiment of this illness. I came to understand that the issue of cancer has meaning not only in the personal context of my life but also in the broader context of the society and world in which we live. Such ways of seeing and working apply to all symptoms and are of essential importance, I believe, to bring to the healing potential of inner work.

I enter a waking dream, an active imagination, to connect again with a figure who has appeared in my inner world. Such a person or image may appear for the purpose of calling attention to a neglected aspect of ourselves. In the Middle Ages, Mary Watkins tells us, "it was a common practice to hold conversations with the soul to ask it questions and to hear answers arising from a source other than consciousness."[1] But it is not so any longer; many of us seem to have forgotten how to pray or meditate or gain access to inner sources other than consciousness. Our culture seems to doubt not only the value but the reality of such aspects of Self, or Divine, or the interface between the two.

I move into stillness and wait to meet with Soul Woman, as she has called herself, the woman of my cancer, and our encounter unfolds in my imagination as I picture our meeting. She has appeared to me before, to teach me about the need for learning about silence and stillness, quiet growth, waiting, loosening, searching in the circular maze of inner and outer journeying. She appeared originally as I attempted to circumambulate the reality of cancer, to discover or create meaning in the experience. Watkins suggests that one may be more receptive to visions in a state of illness or depression, the underworld experiences, because "one's energy is drawn away from the objects it usually participates with. One's being is drawn inward and downward," and it is there one becomes open to allowing and encouraging the meeting with the guest.[2]

This day I ask to meet with Soul Woman again; I quiet my mind and rest in stillness and wait. After a while she appears outside, sitting on a bench. I join her, and we sit together in silence. Then our spirits get up and dance together, and when they are finished we lie down under the tree on the grass and rest. We wait. She leads me then to the top of a mountain. There is a temple here, very old and crumbling: the white columns have broken off and weeds have grown up all around it. I wonder whose temple it is, and she answers, *This is the temple of women. You have been worshipping at the wrong temple.* I feel myself acknowledging and answering the deep truth of her words with my tears, and we begin to work to repair the damage to the temple. The columns are restored to their original wholeness by our attention, and we are pleased by the repaired image.

It is a place of whiteness and simplicity: the tall, white, fluted columns of wood hold up the white roof, and the sides are open to sunlight and breeze, the blues of sky and sea, the greens of growing earth. We wear long white robes, simple and comfortable, and we sit on the grass by the temple. Our encounter comes to an end; we sit, and rest, and wait.

We finish much as we began, resting and waiting. I pause for a while after our visit is over, and I take time to let the experience seep deep into my bones and flesh. This is body-knowing she is teaching me, and I know I must slow down my rhythms to let it enter.

I wonder about the images she has brought to me: the broken columns, much like the severed trunk of the tree; the whiteness of temple and robes; the pleasure of resting and the wisdom of waiting; and the central image of the temple of women.

I go to the sand tray to learn more about this temple of women and the other temple, the wrong one, where I have directed my energy. In Jungian work, the sand tray offers another possible place of expression for the contents of psyche. A tray, about the size of a large serving tray, is partially filled with sand which can be shaped and sculpted. There are shelves of symbolic figures and objects which can be placed in the tray in any arrangement. The process offers a place for imagination to be free, for the soul to play as a child plays. What emerges is usually a combination of intentional and sometimes surprising elements, a mix of conscious and unconscious choices. One seems to be pulled to certain objects, often without understanding why. The result is a kind of snapshot of the soul.

As I enter the room, I am surrounded on three sides by shelves of objects. At first I feel overwhelmed by the abundance of options, and then I realize I have to slow down, to quiet my mind, to sense what may be calling to me. I fill two sand trays with things that seem to belong in the two temples and connect them with a rope of small pearls. I step back to let the symbols work in my psyche. It seems most appropriate to honor the process with structure of a less rigid form, and so I let the words arrange themselves more loosely on the page:

I choose the items carefully
or perhaps they choose me;
this temple furnishing
is intricate
and careful
work.

Crystal, first,
all sizes and shapes
for soul seeing through,
and in the center
a crystal jar, placed carefully,
containing
and ordering
everything around it.
Perhaps the word makes meaning;
perhaps meaning births the word.

There are baskets of grain and fruit and a jug of
water,
plenty, for the journey,
for this temple involves a wandering
and a search.
There is a basket of colors
to paint my canvas, if I want,

though mostly my palette
is pencil.

There is a small sailboat
moved only as the wind blows
and a compass
for knowing direction
though it often doesn't work.
One must always wait for the wind
and the messenger.
Perhaps a bird will fly down
carrying a letter
in its beak.

There are the roots of the tree
underground
just barely visible to the eye:
this is a time of root growing,
not a time for leaves.

Eyes look for leaves too soon
and kill the roots.
Rootedness in the earth is what is needed,
rootedness in the feminine
in this temple of women
where there is time
and growth is allowed
in its season.

There is a very old cave
half buried in the earth,
the outside, rough brown rock,
the inside filled with the dancing light of jewels.

Such is the way of women:
the treasure comes from a deep hidden inside
place,
and is old,
very old.

The temple is complete
for this day
though there is an empty space
to remind me
that it can never be fully furnished,
finished,
and must always be visited
again.

She has led me here,
Soul Woman, as she is called,
and stands beside the temple
as I work.
Her eyes are soft,
not the eyes of killing;
she watches
and watches over
me.

A long chain of pearls
connects the temple
with the not-temple:
woman's milk
spilt
in small perfect drops,
tears
chained together
to be worn as a badge.

In the other, the shadow, the wrong temple
reminders from the past, from otherwheres:
heavy food, from a land of scarcity
grown fat with fear,
scales, for weighing and measuring,
a ladder, for climbing high,
trying to find safety, perhaps,
a table with no meal,
a tree with no roots,
a box, wrapped as a present
with nothing
inside,
not a containing, completing emptiness,
just absence,
like a self,
decorated and sold
too easily.
And the eyes,
watching and killing.

From the nothingness of the prostituted treasure
to the waiting for the season of growth,
it is a long journey in a small sailboat,
waiting for the wind,
for the roots to grow,
for the treasure to spill forth from the cave.
Perhaps the bird will never come
or perhaps there will be no message.

The string of pearls,
the milky tears of woman's grief:
her milk
is not enough,

not ever enough.
Like rosary beads
she prays over each one,
each loss,
each grief,
each not enough,
and slowly
very slowly
if the compass works
and the wind blows
and the bird flies
she may journey to the temple
before the roots are dead.
She may reach it in time.

These are messages from psyche in the form of images and symbols, not to be translated into other meanings, but to be held and examined. I wonder what are they about? What are they pointing toward?

I look first at the elements in the wrong temple, those symbols which are not to be included in the temple of women. Some seem to carry themes of what we usually think of as masculine: weighing and measuring, evaluating and judging, eyes which are critical and unaccepting, dangerous to the tender shoots of growth and the beginning roots.

Echoing the dream of the damaged tree, there is a table with no meal and a tree with no roots, as form is valued over substance. There is the appearance of a gift without the giving, the gilding of the exterior at the expense of interior. There is food, but it is food associated with fear of scarcity, fear that there is not enough, will never be enough. It is food of the Great Mother archetype which, when dishonored, may emerge as the obese literalization of her might and power.

What of the items in the temple of women? There is, first of all, crystal for seeing and containing, another image of glass for viewing soul. The jar placed in the center suggests the containing and ordering principles of creativity, enriching all around it.

There are baskets of grain and fruit, food grown from the earth, and a jug of clear water, a feminine image mingling aspects of containing, cleansing, purifying, satisfying. And there are colors to play with, to make art with, to create and make beautiful, not in the sense of gilding the outside but in letting the spirit of play and the richness of the interior emerge in full color.

There is the need for understanding and honoring what is interior, secret, hidden away. There is the sense of allowing rather than forcing the inner treasure to spill forth, shine forth. There is emphasis on waiting, for the wind to blow or the message to appear. There may be use for a compass here, perhaps a kind of masculine instrument to plot and navigate direction, useful when one must understand the maneuvers of tacking, of sailing against the wind in tangential directions to get to where one is eventually to be.

It is breast cancer which has brought me to this temple of women, to learn about worshipping in this place. It has been, and continues to be, a personal journey, one that has specific implications and meanings for me, but I have wondered if it may be meaningful to other women. I was amazed recently when a friend who had read an early version of this book told me she had heard the identical words in a dream some years ago: "you have been worshipping at the wrong temple." I was stunned; I felt myself take a deep pause to reflect on such a powerful connection. Have other women received such a summons, such a call for change? Are there many of us who need to learn about worshipping at the temple of women?

I think about ways to envision the issue of breast cancer in the world and specifically in the patriarchal world in which we live.

I take in not only the beauty and growth of springtimes, of trees and stars and a handful of earth, but also pollution and violence. I take in the potentially destructive elements of our society: the competitiveness, the anxiety, the tension. And I take in the attitudes of the patriarchy toward the feminine, attitudes which may be critical, devaluing, limiting, oppressive. I imagine it may be these things, which are foreign and alien to our souls, that may become the lump of breast cancer, the lump of the undissolved.

For a woman in the patriarchy, it may become, I imagine, a lump of silence. It is the unspeakable, the heart's desire she does not yet know and the temple she does not yet acknowledge. I want to ask women, How have you been silenced? How have you been unable or unwilling to find your own voice? How have you felt controlled by money, by power, by the need to serve others, by the desire to be liked, by the image of the feminine woman, by the role of wife and mother, by the standard of the good girl, by the wish to please, by the tyranny of the nice? Have you been blind and deaf to your desires, the longings of your heart?

I don't think it is simply that women have been silenced by men; too easy a trap to fall into, such blaming again gives away the power. But it is perhaps more difficult in our society for a woman to find her voice, her authentic feminine inner woman's voice. It seems so often to be a whisper, or a tentative, questioning, half-formed sentence, or, if more definite, a shrill "bitchy" demand of one who isn't really sure she deserves what she is asking for.

I feel affirmed when I find other women who share some of my meanings of cancer. Lorrie Moore writes of the lump in her breast in her novel, *Anagrams*: "I could feel the lump in my breast rise into my throat, from where perhaps it had fallen to begin with."[3] It is the voice, silenced; perhaps that is where it all begins. The lump in one's throat as one begins to speak, the hesitation, the catch, the pain, is the undissolved, the undissolvable. And then, perhaps, it becomes the lump in the breast, near the heart, the heart pain of not having a voice, of not even knowing the heart's desire. I imagine how such a woman might feel.

Her desires
lie buried under layers of
his choices.

She is disappointed,
not only that she will never get
what she may want
but that she will never even know
what it is.
It is the way of things,
even here,
even now.

She learned long ago
not to want,
to find safety
and strength
in the killing of desire.
It is not so hard any more.

But something stays dead,
she has learned:
a little piece,
a little more each time
stays dead.
Some days she wonders
if she will find the perfect solution,
the ultimate
not
wanting.

Deena Metzger, speaking out of her experience of breast cancer, says it even more forcefully and angrily in *The Book of Hags*: "Every woman I know has been dying of silence."[4] Such killing silence is terrifyingly common, she suggests, as breast cancer is terrifyingly common. In *The Cancer Journals*, Audre Lorde speaks of the need for "the transformation of silence into language and action. . . . I have come to believe over and over again," she says, "that what is most important to me must be spoken, made verbal and shared, even at the risk of having it bruised or misunderstood. That the speaking profits me, beyond any other effect."[5]

Death, as a possibility which is intensely present to the woman with cancer, may serve to heighten the need for breaking silence around the self. "I was going to die," Lorde continues, "if not sooner then later, whether or not I had ever spoken myself. My silences had not protected me. Your silence will not protect you."[6] To speak myself–perhaps that too is worship at the temple of women.

It is Lorde's daughter who answers her fear of speaking herself, just as my daughters have often led me to deeper knowing of self. She says to her mother, "You're never really a whole person if you remain silent, because there's always that one little piece inside of you that wants to be spoken out." She warns further that "if you don't speak it out one day it will just up and punch you in the mouth."[7] Or in the breast, perhaps, I add.

Lorde asks questions I would ask myself, and I would ask of other women. "What are the words you do not yet have: What do you need to say? What are the tyrannies you swallow day by day and attempt to make your own, until you will sicken and die of them, still in silence?"[8] One needs to find the voice beyond fear that can speak the truths for which there are not yet words, to become the voice of the voiceless.

It is crucial to remember that, although transformation is called for, a transformation of silence into language and action, one must take care to honor the image as it appears and not rush to change it into something else. That, paradoxically, is one of the essential elements of worship at the temple of women. It is so easy to think we grasp the meaning of the image too quickly; as Watkins says of our attitudes toward our inner images, "we betray them with our sweet understandings."[9] It is an inner honoring we must give to the image seeking our attention. Watkins cautions further: "When we turn from the image and change our life in the world in terms simply of activity, the image becomes incredibly frustrated because that is not her only world. She did not raise her voice to have us turn further from her."[10]

It will not be enough to cut out the lump in the throat or the lump in the breast, any more than it is enough to eradicate the symptom or the symptom bearer. Wisdom must come from the lump itself, which can, if honored, lead one to the right temple. Moore speaks for many women with breast cancer when she writes: "The lump was not simply a focal point for my self-pity; it was also a battery propelling me, strengthening me–my very own appointment with death. It anchored and deepened me like a secret."[11]

Not every woman has a lump in the breast, but I believe many women are suffering from not having a voice, from not worshipping at the temple of women. It is not enough to cut out what will not dissolve in one's being; one must learn to follow it to the temple. What is this temple to which we have been summoned? I think of it as the place of women, but it is both more and less than that. To name it is inadequate to the image, as always, but perhaps useful in the struggle to understand meaning. It is for and about what we usually think of as feminine values. For me, it is a deeper call to body, to soul, to Self. It is about more fully trusting my instincts, honoring my truths, giving voice to my reality. It is about turning inward for guidance and creativity. It is about making time and space to pray and play.

The work is never completed, but it can be started. Just as I left a space in one corner of the temple to honor the essential quality of never-finished-ness, so the image must be summoned again and again, so the temple must be visited again and again. And so the metaphor continues to emerge, to change, to fill out. As the image of the waking dream is to be allowed to grow and change, so with the metaphor. The lump of cancer, the lump of the undissolved, the lump of silence, becomes yet one more metaphor: the lump of clay, to be worked and reworked, again and again, never completed, always becoming.

INTERLUDE

Wording the Process

I write in pencil
so I can work the words;
like clay,
they must not harden
too soon.

One cannot write poetry at a computer.
Poetry must be made by hand,
pencil and paper,
the wood of a tree
worked.
Words written,
looked at,
listened to,
felt,
changed.

Erasures and smudges are good.
Lurches and stumbling are necessary.
This is not to be a casual stroll in the park.

7

A Blaze for the Journey

I often think that I have not yet been ill enough to know how to live.

—Arthur Frank, *At the Will of the Body*

ANY JOURNEY INTO the unknown can be dangerous and terrifying; one fears getting lost forever and never being able to find the way back to the known, the safe, the comfortable. A tribe in Africa has a ritual for the beginning of such a journey: a blaze or mark is cut into a tree at the very edge of the known world, the place where it interfaces with the unknown. Such a blaze is made so the hunter can venture into new territory and still be able to find his way back to the familiar safety of the village.[1]

The ritual of the blaze thus becomes the metaphor for metaphor: it is the two-sided image cut precisely at the edge of the familiar territory, facing toward both the known and the unknown.[2] It is metaphor that can carry us to the edge of the unknown and point us in the direction of the new area that needs to be explored.

Cancer has been such a blaze for me. Although the scar was not cut by my own hand, it has become a blaze through the process of making meaning and creating metaphor from a physical reality. Cut at the edge of my area of safety and comfort, it has served to signal my threshold to the unknown, to the unconscious, to the feared, and ultimately to death. I imagine it to be the mark between obligation and desire, between convention and creativity, between conscious and unconscious, between ego and Self.

My blaze, breast cancer, marks the growing edge. A physical bodily scar never goes away and keeps changing throughout a lifetime. What is true of a visible scar may also be true, I believe, of an invisible scar, an inner blaze: it never disappears and constantly keeps changing, underlining the aspect of process in life and in consciousness and calling for change and growth. My external scar seemed to pull in on itself, reflecting the change in my inner world as it pulled in and deepened.

One of the effects of the blaze of cancer is to turn me in other directions. I imagine the blaze was cut by a part of myself needing to grow in a certain direction, needing to explore new territory. She may be a hunter of another kind of reality. She may need to search for meaning deeper in the forest; she may have a hunger for a food that cannot be found within the confines of the village. She may need to wander simply for the sake of wandering, to venture away from the safe and the conventional because it is too restricting. And she may need to go beyond the fear to begin to live differently, without even knowing what that means.

Grace Butcher sketches an image of a woman afraid, who looks just beyond the edge of her fear and wonders, "What would you do now if you were not afraid?" She imagines an answer coming from the person who "lives just outside all her boundaries and constantly calls her to come over, come over."[3] I like this image of a self who lives on the other side of the blaze, who lives just outside my boundaries of fear, and who can speak to me and summon me to cross the line of the known, the safe. She may be the one who etched the blaze of cancer on the tree in which we both live, who knew, even when I did not, what was needed.

As living scar tissue keeps changing, the blaze of cancer can pull me to many different unknown territories. Beginning with the circumference of a circle, one drawn perhaps too tight and close around my world of safe and proper, it seemed to be able to move anywhere around the perimeter. Again I became aware of the unpredictable growth pattern: as edges were bumped out here and there, the circle became misshapen. Still perhaps a vaguely rounded shape, balanced by a foray first in one direction, then another, then another, it now looks more like the irregular edges of cellular growth. It reminds me of a garden without precise lines and sharp edges, arranged in patterns that are looser and more freely etched.

One of the possible edges marked by a blaze is the line between ego and Self. Erich Fromm's work on the distinctions between "having" and "being" offer us a way of thinking about ego and Self. The having mode, according to Fromm, focuses on acquisition: "The attitude inherent in consumerism is that of swallowing the whole world."[4] One's identity is based on the philosophy of consumerism: in the having mode, one's worth equates to what one has or what one consumes. In this mode, explains Fromm, people experience themselves as a commodity to be marketed and sold. They "prepare" themselves for the important meeting and tally their assets of successes, social status, connections, appearance, and personality; they "mentally balance their worth" and "display their wares."[5]

Such is the mode of ego. Ego lives within the village and is concerned with safety and having: the acquisition of things is, I believe, one of the ways in which ego attempts to feel safe. Ego is concerned with fortifying its position and surrounding itself with things to protect itself; objects, money, achievements, and successes can all become barricades around the village.

Self is much more the lone hunter who ventures off into the forest, traveling alone, carrying little, unprotected, looking less for safety than for truth and authenticity. It knows there is no safety in things and is more interested in a different kind of having.

Self understands the day of Shabbat as a true day of rest, a time dedicated to "the reestablishment of complete harmony between human beings and between them and nature."[6] The Shabbat, therefore, is "a day of joy because on that day one is fully oneself," and this is the treasure sought by Self.[7]

Self understands inner poverty as that which is embraced by one who "wants nothing, knows nothing, and has nothing."[8] This entity is the Buddha who leaves all possessions to live a life of nonattachment, the Christ who "had nothing and–in the eyes of the world–is nothing, yet who acts out of the fullness of his love for all human beings."[9] And yet Self understands the paradox of such poverty and knows when one is rich in the "powers of . . . love, of artistic and intellectual creation, all essential powers grow through the process of being expressed. What is spent is not lost, but on the contrary, what is kept is lost."[10]

Having, for Self, is different from the acquisitive drive of the ego: it is a kind of being-having. Georgia O'Keeffe seemed to be speaking about this different kind of having when she said about Pedernal, the mountain she painted again and again, "God told me if I painted it often enough, I could have it."[11] This is the kind of having the Self is interested in, not about possessing the other but about having a relationship with the other, whether the other is a person or an object. If we approach an experience with openness and freedom and respect, it becomes ours in this way of relationship.

It is a different kind of having, this having that is accomplished through relationship, either through intimacy with another person or through the creation of art. It involves, I believe, an understanding that we are not separate entities, cut off from each other and from nature. This is what Thich Nhat Hanh speaks about when he coined the term *interbeing*.[12] He describes how things *inter-are* with each other: everything connects with and depends upon everything else. "We cannot just be by ourselves alone," he says; "we have to inter-be with every other thing." He uses an example of roses and garbage, which we usually judge so differently, but which are closely connected. The blooming rose withers and decays, becoming garbage in a matter of a few days, and garbage can be used as fertilizer to grow another rose.[13]

This kind of having, whether it be of mountains, visions, or relationships, involves a loosening. It is having with an open palm, not a closed, grasping fist. It is having without strings, without expectations. It means painting the mountain so many times that one forms an intimate connection with it, that mountain and self become part of each other, which is the only real and lasting and meaningful kind of having. And it means finishing the painting or the piece of writing simply because it is essential to finish it, because there is a completeness in the honoring of the vision, even if no one else will ever see it.

In relationships, such a notion of having means valuing the intimacy that occurs between people as it happens, without trying to make it other than what it is, without strings, without expectations. It is the opposite, as Fromm suggests, of wanting to possess the other. It is, again, the open hand. May Sarton writes, in *Journal of a Solitude*, "Perhaps the greatest gift we can give to another human being is detachment. Attachment, even that which imagines it is selfless, always lays some burden on the other person."[14] To be in intimate relationship without laying a burden on the other is, I believe, the being way of relating to the other.

The gift given with the open hand is what is called in some Native American traditions one's "giveaway." As one is given a certain talent, one is also under a certain obligation to develop and share it with others. It has become a personal issue. I was asked once by a colleague if he could give something I had written on breast cancer to a client who was experiencing the same disease. It was a very personal and meaningful piece to me, and I felt somewhat reluctant, at first, to put it in the hands of someone I didn't know.

As I was considering my decision, I remembered a story Lynn Andrews relates in one of her books, where she is told by her Native American guide to tie a copy of her latest book onto a nearby tree so that any traveler who passes by could take it. When I recalled this image of a giveaway, I decided to give my writing to the unknown reader on my path. Even though I don't know anything about the woman who read my words, I feel a connection to her, not only through the cancer we both have experienced, but by the ribbon tying the gift. It is the ribbon that speaks to the inter-are of the world and not the strings so often connected to what is not freely given.

In searching for an image that suggests these qualities of being and the sense of inter-are, I recall the image of the tree. It has been for me an image of self and soul; how appropriate that it also speaks to the extension of self and soul into the world. The tree, which is the place where the blaze is cut, and the place where the giveaway is tied, becomes my image of inter-are.

Cancer has become a blaze for me. Like the scar cut on the tree of self, it has called me to come over, come over. It has called me first of all to recognize and honor the connectedness imaged by the tree, the inter-are of all being. As the tree has its roots in the earth and reaches up to the sun with its leaves, so I too am a being of earth and sky. I have begun to learn to honor both my rootedness in the earth, in the feminine, in soul, and my reaching toward sky, toward spirit.

I continue to watch for and honor any movement from a position of ego to a position of Self. The steps are small at first, as the leaf begins to unfurl from the bud. I have realized anew the importance of writing, not for approval or recognition from anyone else, but as a way of honoring my vision. It is of essential importance to put the final brushstroke on the painting, whether or not it is ever seen by another. And I have also realized, paradoxically, the importance of offering the giveaway to another who may walk along the path I have taken. It is not to be secreted away in the attic but shared with others who may walk the same path.

Cancer has been the metaphor that has led me to metaphor, to learn to live in the metaphor. It has been the blaze that has taken me deeper into the forest, to explore the ancient caves and hunt for the treasure. It has taken me within and down to my inner realities and has taught me about the imaginal in new ways. Dreams and waking dreams have become more important, and the voices of the gods are heard both within and without. It is the blaze, the metaphor, that can lead us deep into the forest to hunt for what we need.

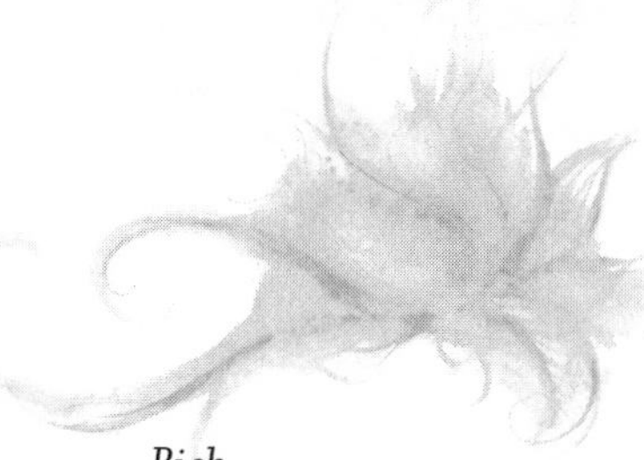

Rich

Riches:
the society lady on Saturday night
well-fed and ornamented,
face painted over,
waiting
to be amused.

Richness:
the hymn on a Sunday morning
sung by a full choir and congregation,
the church, a series of vaults and spires,
carved, colored,
lofting high,
the space enclosed,
sacred and deep.
Outside
the sun is still warm
but the light begins to whisper
of winter.

Rich:
the song
and the silence
just after.

8

The Journey Continues

Which parts of myself are too greedy, which selves go hungry, wither and die?

—Deena Metzger, *Tree*

ONE OF THE LAST cancerous lumps I have had to confront is the lump of fear. I had some scares in the years following my original diagnosis: there were tests on several occasions that indicated possible recurrence of the disease, and I had to live with that possibility each time until further testing concluded there was no recurrence.

On one occasion, an analysis of a needle biopsy indicated there were cancer cells present again in the same breast. I decided I would have a mastectomy a few days later, at the same time as a previously scheduled procedure to extract bone marrow for storage and use in case the cancer metastasized. If that occurred, it would require a more severe form of chemotherapy, possible only with some of my own harvested "clean" bone marrow which could then be given back to me. I agreed to the mastectomy at the same time but asked the surgeon to do a thorough biopsy of the site and confirm the presence of cancerous cells before proceeding.

It turned out there was no evidence of any malignancy. My

husband told me later that the surgeon had done multiple frozen sections to look for cancer cells and had come out after each one to tell him there was no evidence of disease. The medical staff understood the outcome as a rare occurrence of a misreading of the first results, due probably to the presence of scar tissue. I understood it as a miracle, however it could be explained, and I try to remember to be thankful daily for the miracle of life.

So it has not been easy to go back into the realities of cancer in order to write about it. I have experienced many levels of fear. I have been afraid to look too intensely at all the realities I had endured: afraid to remember too closely, and afraid I have not remembered closely enough. I fear that I haven't been faithful to the lessons of cancer, that I haven't lived fully enough, haven't risked enough, haven't grown enough. I fear that I play it too safe. I fear that I don't live what I have learned, or should have learned. I fear that I am not grateful enough, that I take life and health and relationships and all the gifts I have too much for granted.

Some of the issues I have wrestled with have come in the guises of time and space. Time has changed since cancer. Maybe in the second half of life time changes anyway, but cancer seems to have increased the speed of change. I struggle with questions of how to spend time most fruitfully. I have trouble "passing" time in ways that do not nourish the soul. But sometimes "wasting" time is the most soulful expression of self. How to balance time for doing and time for being? How to find time for connection with others and also with the depths within myself and for creative expression of my imaginal reality? The lessons of cancer continue to demand growth. I remember writing about the conflict:

> Urgency robs time's pleasures.
>
> I am an addict,
> desire never satisfied,

except
when I stop
to savor
the spaciousness
of dawn.

The lump of fear was at times paralyzing. I did nothing sometimes, or stayed so busy I didn't have time to contemplate deeper realities and then crashed into exhausted periods of doing nothing again. I neglected my body, even as I wrote about attending to its rhythms, its needs.

It seemed as if the prospect of writing, like cancer, was itself a threat to life. Having survived, so far, I did not welcome what felt like the constricting and demanding task of writing. For a long time I struggled with the dilemma, trying to force myself to write and vigorously resisting, immobilized in a trap of my own making. I knew the conflict was poisoning my life, and I continued to struggle with questions about wasting time and using time and enjoying time, but I could not find a resolution. I finally realized I wanted to let go of the demand and see what that freedom felt like, but I found that something pulled me back to the writing.

After a long time of inner work and preparation, I was granted a moment of grace that helped me see things differently. A quote I came across from Rabbi Tarfon transformed my struggle: "It is not required of you that you complete the task but neither are you free to abandon it."[1] The goal changed: I had to move from focusing on the product to focusing on the process. I had to be faithful to the task and yet not be attached to the outcome. I felt a loosening of the familiar death grip in my hand and in my life.

I finally gave myself permission to rest, to enjoy leisure. One of the most terrifying realizations was that some part of me, the part that desperately wanted to avoid the inner struggle, was almost wishing for a recurrence of cancer; then I would not have to address the task or the conflict. It was just barely conscious, but when I heard whispers of it in myself, I was very frightened. I have realized one of the crucial questions in this struggle is: What would a return of cancer allow me to ignore? I wonder if other women have ever heard such a whisper, have ever thought about what difficulties would just go away if cancer returned. Does such a thought, barely under the radar of consciousness, have a negative effect on the immune system? I believe it does. Once it can be identified and faced directly, it can be changed.

I am usually very efficient, sometimes killingly efficient. Because time is so precious, I want to use it well. But the very attempt to use it well is itself often a misuse of time. I have made efficiency a god sometimes in place of leisure and joy. To attempt to control time destroys spontaneity; to hold on too tightly as time slips quickly away is killing to the life process itself. I recalled Judith Duerk's statement that illness gives permission to rest, and I vowed to give it to myself without the necessity of illness. I tried to learn to have a different relationship with time.

> Morning woke me
> early
> today.
> Unlike the shrill demand
> of the clock
> insisting on schedule and task,
> it was the subtle invitation of cool sunlight,
> not yet harsh and bleaching,
> the beckoning of leaves barely moving,
> the promise of stillness and solitude.
>
> It was Saturday
> in fact and feeling.

Space is another issue I have engaged in battle. The need for psychic space has had echoes in the need for space in the external world. I recall some lines of poetry I wrote:

It is not
enough
any more
to have a room of my own;
I need the whole house empty.
The longing
grows
like cancer.

Like cancer
which grew so insistently in my breast
demanding
too much space
near my heart,
uncontainable,
the desire grows.

Womanbreast and womanheart,
trained early toward the other:
I have never learned to close my ear
to the footsteps outside my door.

So what I long for is space,
room to dance naked
with no unwanted gaze,
time to sit alone
and breathe the silence.

This I have learned from cancer:

I am no longer willing
to be contained
by reasonable limits.
I want the whole house
and more.

I realize I still struggle with the conflicting pulls of interiority and external relationships. I know, theoretically and deeply within myself, that I have to have time and space and solitude for connection to myself in order to be able to connect more deeply with others. I know also that intimacy with others is connected to, not opposed to, intimacy with self. But there are often difficult choices. External demands and expectations from others are somewhat more easily dealt with. I am no longer willing to do the conventional thing for the sake of form; it is not a good enough reason any more.

The choice becomes more difficult, however, when a variety of opposing options are all desirable. I want to have more time for leisure and play, and I also want to honor with consistency and faithfulness the work I do with clients. I need to clear spaces of time for myself to meander through inner landscapes and write of the realities I encounter there, and I also want to spend more time with family and friends. Balance sometimes seems difficult to achieve. And sometimes I want not to be balanced but to be able to allow myself to be consumed by whatever psyche longs for.

One of the paradoxical gifts of breast cancer is that living in the shadow of death makes life sweeter, more compelling, more intense. If we avoid what we are called to, we pay the price. But when we follow the calling, stumbling through the dark, labyrinthine ways psyche seems to prefer, we gain the reward.

I sometimes think of cancer as a house where I used to live, one which holds terrors for me and which I fear to enter again. I recall a dream about a house, about revisiting the house I lived in as a child. There are other people living in the house now; I ask if I can look through it, and they let me in. I explore the first floor, especially the kitchen. Then I go upstairs, using the main stairs, and check to see if there are still back stairs from the kitchen to the landing. At the top of the stairs, unlike the external reality of the historical past, is my parents' bedroom. It is painted red now, and an old roof patio is opened up as part of the room. The whole house seems larger and nicer than I remember.

I try to enter the dream as I might enter this literal house to look around and see what I can find, what it feels like, what I experience and remember and imagine. The dream takes me back to a childhood home and offers me the opportunity to look at it from a different perspective. I am especially drawn to the kitchen, the place of cooking and transforming of matter. I remember pleasant family breakfasts eaten there on weekends, and I remember how it was my task to make weekday breakfasts of bacon and eggs for my family when my mother was getting ready to go to work. There is a sense of the heightened ambivalence I experienced in my family in the mix of memories, happiness and sadness entwined in the various recollections.

I see my parents' room differently now, the dream tells me: it is red, a vivid color of warmth, intensity, even passion. And it has been opened up, enlarged, with the addition of what used to be a sunroof. Things appear larger, even nicer than I remember them. I remember the earlier dream about my parents' house in which the addition of a room killed the tree that was close to the circular staircase. In that dream, I sat with my family as if to eat dinner, but there was no food present. I was a daughter among other daughters of my parents; there was sadness because of abuse by the masculine to the feminine, but my sadness was met by irrelevance from my parents.

I realize again that the abuse of the feminine by the masculine continues in my psyche in the form of an inner critic. I have experienced it most clearly in my work on this project, but as always, the issues revolving around cancer are about my life as a whole. I strain to impose too much linear order on the meandering organic nature of feminine growth. I am critical of my attempts at creativity and convince myself they are worthless. I label, I judge, I criticize, I devalue. I push myself instead of listening to my body's rhythms; I paralyze myself with demands and deadlines and feel guilt when they are not met.

I recognize the need to acknowledge such an inner voice and separate myself from it as a way of loosening its grip on me. In my battle with the inner masculine attacker, he has been winning this skirmish. Trying to fight him with his own weapons hasn't worked, and I have exhausted myself in the attempt. The frontal attack has not gotten me where I want to be; perhaps, as the dream suggests, I should use the back stairs to sneak around behind the scenes when he isn't looking. In the dream, I use the front stairs, but I check to see if the back stairs are still there. I need to be able to move unseen from the kitchen, where something may be cooking, transforming, to the bedroom, which is now red. There is a more direct line of access between the two than that which existed in reality. Something is cooking, something is heating up, reddening.

I think of my associations to red, a color I don't often wear or want around me: it is too vivid, too bright, too much. I prefer paler, more subtle shadings. But there it is, whether I prefer it or not. Perhaps the ego-alien color is there to lead me away from habitual ego perceptions and patterns, away from the historical past. Some new possibility may be presenting itself, symbolized as a red parental bedroom, larger and nicer than I remembered. Perhaps the room for my own inner couple, the masculine and feminine aspects within me, has become more spacious and is able to incorporate more from the outside.

I think of the link between kitchen and bedroom as a

transformative potential. I went through many stages in my reaction to and work with cancer: from the blackness, in the depths of depression and darkness and desolation, to the silver-white experience of lunar consciousness associated with feminine interiority, and then to the red-gold brightness associated with striving masculine solar consciousness. The dream suggests that what was a sunroof is now incorporated into the bedroom of the couple. Solar consciousness, roof high, once separate and outside, is now being integrated inside the room to accommodate both masculine and feminine in the container of their union.

One of the tasks I presently face is finding the place of intensity and passion at the top of my own stairs and letting it expand to include even the rooftop terrace. Perhaps the extra room which killed the roots of the tree in the first dream is imaged here as an outside place that has been incorporated into the inside.

I have delved deeply into lunar consciousness around the issues of cancer and let them resonate within me. I have birthed personal images and nursed them into a fullness of growth. I have grappled with issues of feminine consciousness, both personal and cultural: of respecting and valuing the interior feminine space and silence which is life giving, and of battling the distance and silence imposed on women by others and by themselves in a patriarchal culture. I have struggled with issues of the body and sought to honor its rhythms and wisdom. I think I was finally afraid to try to translate such deeply important feminine truths into the masculine form of structured composition. I was afraid of doing damage to them, to force a Procrustean reshaping of nonlinear truths into linear containers. I was afraid of more masculine abuse.

And so, paradoxically, I became the abuser, again. I tried to make myself reshape the material on demand, and I tried equally hard to resist the effort. The result was often, as I have said, paralysis. No wonder I had to check to see if the back stairs were still there, even as I used the front stairs to go up. Part of me realized this couldn't continue to be a frontal attack. And part of me realized it was time to incorporate the sunroof and the reddening of solar consciousness, but not in an aggressive and attacking mode. It is to be incorporated and included in the red room which is so much larger and nicer now and can include and contain the sunroof and redness of passion, of life.

I was afraid of bringing my writing about cancer into the house where I live; I was afraid that, like cancer, it would take over and choke the pleasure out of my life. On the one hand, I wanted to let it take me over, to submit to the red passion calling me to grapple with it. And on the other hand, I was terrified it would grow like a noxious weed and take over the entire garden of my life. And so I created the very thing I most feared. Anne Sexton quotes a line from Saul Bellow: "Live or die, but don't poison everything."[2] I was allowing the demand to write about cancer to poison everything and the struggle with the animus forces became paralyzingly toxic. The life-and-death struggle with cancer became the life-and-death struggle with writing about cancer.

Clarissa Pinkola Estés writes of the inner critic in her popular book, *Women Who Run with the Wolves.* "Often the creative life is slowed or stopped because something in the psyche has a very low opinion of us, and we are down there groveling at its feet."[3] She exhorts us to "take ourselves, our ideas, our art, far more seriously than we have done before," and she blames our failures to do so on "breaks in matrilineal succor . . . over many generations."[4] The widespread popularity of this book may confirm the pervasiveness of this issue of failed creativity for women and the battle with the critical inner figure to whom we all too often continue to submit.

When I was finally able to see again what was happening, I found a metaphor that allowed me to continue writing. I became a quilt maker, as women have always been. I took the quilt pieces I had already made, kept some and discarded some, and continued to create more quilt pieces from the scraps of material of my life. There were different colors and fabrics and shapes. Some of the fabric pieces were from the work of others who had addressed this topic and whose insights resonated with my truths. Some were old pieces and some were new. I had to be able to work on fashioning each piece without worrying beforehand where exactly it would fit into the finished quilt. It was a difficult process to sustain the creation of such pieces over a long period of time without the sense of how they would all fit together. Some eventually didn't fit and had to be discarded; others looked as if they wouldn't fit, but I found space for them.

I wasn't able to work until I found the metaphor, the quilt making that honors the way women work. And even then the inner critic wasn't quite convinced. *Those quilt pieces*, he seemed to say, *aren't symmetrical: they are different sizes and shapes and don't match. How will you make anything valuable of such random pieces?* Then I saw a quilt hanging in a friend's home, an incredible work of brightly hued, irregularly shaped pieces of fabric. It combined elements of East and West, honoring traditional patterns and creating new colors and shapes. It imaged the possibility of my own final product, and then I was able to create it.

I remember another dream, one of the most compelling I have ever had, that speaks again to the issue of an inner domineering masculine figure. In the dream, a friend is dying. I am with her at her house, a beautiful rustic cabin in the mountains, and I want to take her to see a redbud tree in the afternoon light. We have to drive to see it, and we are going to take an open jeep for the trip. I intend to drive her there, but suddenly a man is in the driver's seat and my friend and I are in the back of the car. I feel great sadness that I am not steering my own life. In waking life, I longed for such a simple cabin; somehow in the dream I felt I would never be able to have it.

Images of tree and house, repeated from earlier dreams, move again through the spiral of psyche. This time the tree is a compelling image which draws me to it in the magic and specificity of the afternoon light. In the afternoon of my life, I am entranced by the beauty of this particularized image of a single redbud tree. It draws me, and as I carry the dream image with me, I feel the continual longing of my soul for this very singular image. The dream is full of pathos, with the sadness of my friend dying, the unfinished trip to see the redbud tree, and the felt loss of the possibility of finding and having the special cabin in the mountains.

The loftiness of the mountains is suggestive to me of masculine spirit. My dying friend is a woman, and I want to drive the car to take her to see the redbud tree. But there is a man in the driver's seat, a man whom I know, who typifies an ordered, linear, lofty, logos-centered approach to life. I felt dismay when I saw him in the driver's seat of my dream car, just as I felt dismay at sensing I would never get the cabin in the woods I so desired.

My friend in the dream is a writer; she signals, I think, the dying state of my own inner writer. The dream occurred at a time when I couldn't write, when I felt a kind of paralysis. Writing carries for me an access to Self. It is one strong way of working with the ego-Self connection between the more conscious ego and the more unconscious aspects of psyche encompassed and centered by the concept of Self. The writer was dying, and the masculine was in the driver's seat. I didn't know if we ever got to the beautiful feminine image of the redbud tree in the soft light of the afternoon of the day, of life.

Dying friend, dying day, dying hopes. The dream both terrified me and called me very strongly to become aware of the realities it expressed. As I wrestled with the implications of this dream over a period of time, I realized I had again let the driving, linear masculine take over both in the process of the writing and in the journey of my life. I was letting the writer die, and I wasn't getting her to the redbud tree. The kind of writing suggested by the call of the redbud tree is poetic, imaginal, feminine, soulful. Whether in the form of poetry or prose or keeping a journal, it elicits a connection with the interior depths that are accessed in the process of the doing. And I was ignoring what I should have been honoring.

> The word
> aches for birth,
> strains
> to break through the crust
> of consciousness,
> demanding life.
>
> Too often
> I deny it breath;
> mired in sludge,
> I turn my face away
> and smile
> at what we usually call
> reality.

Again, it is not so much about getting to the goal of the journey as it is about the journey itself. It is not as important to get to the redbud tree as it is to go in search of it, to honor the longing of soul as it calls to a particular image. It is not as important to have a mountain cabin as it is to find the place of quiet and retreat within myself.

It is the journey and not the destination that is the value of soul. I think of the poem "Ithaka" by C. P. Cavafy, which speaks of the mythic travels of Odysseus. Ithaka is the goal, the compelling end point of the voyage, but the poet describes the true value of the journey as the journey itself. Ithaka is the ultimate destination but not the ultimate value. What will make one rich is not the achievement of that final goal but the sum of all the experiences along the way. "Ithaka gave you the marvelous journey. / Without her you wouldn't have set out. / She has nothing left to give you now."[5]

Breast cancer has given me that marvelous journey. As a physical reality, it was the beginning of my journey and propelled me forward; as a symbolic reality, it was the end point of the journey that called me to new depths. The voyage has been a long one and has included getting graduate degrees in psychology and training as a Jungian analyst, all valuable credentials. But the more important aspects of the journey involve inner exploration and growth and deepening. Culminating in this book, it represents more than twenty years of experience, learning, introspection, writing.

Like Ithaka, the redbud tree called me on a journey, the meandering quest that is valued by soul. Interesting that the redbud blooms in early spring, a first burst of beautiful color after a long and gray winter. It is a fragile and ephemeral blossoming, short-lived, fleeting. After the blooms disappear, large green leaves unfurl to provide a broad canopy of shade throughout the heat of summer. I often sit in the morning under the one in our yard and enjoy a first mug of coffee and some quiet time.

The redbud tree that was the goal of my dream was calling to me in the afternoon light. Paradoxically, the image contains both the early blooming of spring and the late afternoon of a visit. It is perhaps in the afternoon of life that I am called, again, to the rebirth of a new spring. But there is that warning: I can't get there with the male energy in the driver's seat. I love the gentle, delicate image that calls to be honored, another underlining of the temple of the feminine that so strongly summons me. I must remember: in writing, it is the creative process, not the product, that leads me to soul connection. In life, it is about finding the place of silence and simplicity within myself.

I have learned the lesson of process in other ways as well. When I became interested in photography some years ago, I found myself drawn to taking pictures of the natural world: fresh snow on a pine branch, the morning sun silhouetting the outline of a new green leaf, a swirl of daffodils around the trunk of a tree. I captured a red flash of a cardinal sitting on a bare winter branch and a butterfly poised on a purple blossom. I photographed the first snowdrops blooming in the early spring and a single burgundy leaf fallen on the ground in autumn. I moved in closer and closer to a single flower or a seed pod. I enjoyed some of the results and happily framed and hung the images where I could see them often. I made calendars with some of the scenes so I could share them with family and friends, and I made note cards to send messages in the old-fashioned way, handwritten and mailed in actual envelopes. But I realized along the way that the most important result that I gained from taking pictures was learning to see in new ways: to see more intensely, to observe more closely, to notice and appreciate the small displays of beauty that I had so easily overlooked.

The redbud tree was the goal for the journey and the journey itself, just as the work of individuation is the becoming of oneself. It requires the marriage of male and female, of masculine and feminine within oneself. Through this work I learned I have to be both Odysseus, the adventurer who roamed the world and ended up where he had started, and Penelope, faithful spouse, who stayed at home, weaving her work by day and unraveling it by night. Just as Self is both the circumference and the center of psyche, one must both expand and wander and also hold true to the essential center of oneself.

INTERLUDE

December

December should be a time of waiting,
of preparing the silence,
of moving to the still point
within,
of remembering
the story and the stories
of birth
and love.

Nature teaches us how
if we listen through the noise
to the quiet.
Snow falls silently white
and makes a blanket of hush
to soften the earth.
Bare branches of maple
silhouette against the pale liquid
of winter sun
so that we may better see
the flash of scarlet bird.

The earth darkens.
It is the time of longest night
and deepest chill,
sometimes bone deep;
it moves us toward the light and warmth
of morning sun
and evening fire.

December should be a time
of following the star.
I remember the one in Bethlehem
ages old,
and I remember the one I carry near my heart:
the scar star,
stellated, they say,
focusing the pattern of my life,
pulling me to its center.

December should be a time of waiting
but I rush and flurry;
December should be a time of stillness
but the lists jangle.
There was no room at the inn;
there is no room within.
The silence of the star calls
urgently.
It is already
December.

Final Thoughts

Have you lived passionately, made music, given freely, prayed extravagantly, created useless beauty, attempted spontaneous kindness, pondered deeply, shaped gently what you touched, have you loved beauty?

—W. Paul Jones, *A Table in the Desert*

IT HAS BEEN twenty-six years now since I was diagnosed with cancer. I have lived with the possibility of recurrence for all those years, punctuated by annual mammograms and checkups with my oncologist. Some years the stress was more intense than others: when I was called back for more mammogram pictures or when I needed a core needle biopsy to analyze suspicious growth. One year I was out of town with my two daughters when I received the news that the annual results showed suspected cancer growth. I remember we made a fire on the beach and roasted marshmallows for s'mores and cried and even laughed together. It is a sweet memory now of a time of connection even through the pain.

The annual checkups were always difficult. I remember once when I was having a routine test of some kind, the medical technician touched my arm in a gesture of empathy or support, and I dissolved into tears. Although my response was partly a release of tension, I think it was mostly a deep appreciation of the simple but moving expression of human connection and care. It is my hope that these words may forge such a connection with others who have shared this difficult journey, even through the pain.

Cancer and aging have collaborated to continue to teach me how to live more fully, more deeply, more authentically. Although there are many negative aspects connected with a diagnosis of cancer, I have found that the experience of illness does magnify the joy to be found in simple experiences. One of my friends said recently she has noticed that people who have had cancer don't expect life to be perfect. I think those of us who have been touched by the disease and the threat of death are able to be grateful for daily gifts and blessings even when things are not perfect.

I have learned to savor and feel gratitude for the small and ordinary moments of life. Having a morning cup of coffee outside when the weather is nice or an evening glass of wine with my husband as we watch the sunset and talk about our memories and dreams. Watching the change of seasons: the crisp air and deep colors of fall, the first magical snowfall of winter, the early bulbs pushing up to meet the warmth of spring, the longer and slower green days of summer. Being able to take a walk and ride a bike and go to an exercise class. Taking a nap on a lazy afternoon and getting lost in a good book at any time. Hearing the piercing call of a loon across a lake and the soft summons of a dove announcing the dawn. Sharing laughter with grandchildren and tears with friends who face into pain and loss. Enjoying good conversations that go beneath the superficiality of conventional exchange. Playing with photography and painting, not only for the fun of creativity but also for the lessons of noticing and appreciating beauty everywhere. Seeing the redbud tree in the afternoon light.

I am grateful, too, for the gift of being able to share the journeys of my clients over the years as they walked their own paths of individuation. I have worked with some amazing women and have learned much from them. They have inspired me with their commitment to inner work, to looking deeply into their own lives and issues. Because of my own underworld experiences, I think I have been better able to accompany the sometimes painful journeys of others. I have felt myself to be an advocate for their souls, and I have felt honored to be trusted to create a safe and secure container for the work.

I keep a piece of art in my therapy office that embodies for me an image of an essential aspect of the work of inner exploration, the becoming of oneself more fully and richly and completely. Created by the artist Margeaux Klein, it is named *The Only Witness*. The story of its genesis is as compelling as the piece itself. Some years ago, Margeaux bought a hundred-year-old schoolhouse to serve as both home and studio and discovered dozens of old books in the basement of the building. As she began to work with them to create the art she made, they became the central concepts of her work. The book became an image of self, the story of oneself, dragged up from the basement and reclaimed, remembered, re-created.

The book as she worked with it was sometimes made illegible, sometimes closed tightly, sometimes put inside a secure container. In the piece in my office, a small book is open, its pages blackened and unreadable. Cut into the pages on one side is a hollowed out space; on the other side is attached a small rectangular shape that fits precisely into the space and would become invisible if closed. The book is placed in a box which can close around it and hide it entirely. The box and the book are both blackened with some material that rubs off on the hands of anyone who touches them.

Like a true symbol which cannot be reduced to one meaning, this piece of art carries many layers of meaning: the text of oneself, often difficult or impossible to understand, sometimes closed tightly around a secret, sometimes contained, sometimes concealed; appearing in images found or unbidden; affecting and infecting others, leaving its mark on those who touch it and are touched by it; carrying the ambivalence of wanting to be known and wanting to be hidden. And always there is the powerful statement that there is only one who has had the experience, who knows from inside, who embodies the story–the only witness.

Each of us is the only witness to our own story, to the deepest hidden truth of ourselves, the fears and failures and hopes and treasures. We need to learn how to read the text, and we must be willing to look deep within, even when it means rummaging in the basement for whatever lurks there, even when it means being marked by touching the truth.

When I think of being a witness to our journeys of self-discovery, I think of the Greek goddess Hecate, the carrier of crone wisdom. In the story of the underworld experience of Persephone, it is Hecate who hears her cries for help. She listens from inside her cave, the myth tells us, and waits in silence for a time before acting. We need to be there when we listen and wait, I think, in the cave, in the dark silence. Even as the Persephone part of ourselves is enduring an underworld experience, we need also to be Hecate and wait and listen to soul and body for the wisdom of their teachings. We need to be able to hear and acknowledge our own cries for help and be willing to learn the language of the unconscious, to learn to read the text of story.

It is a painful experience to be yanked out of a comfortable upper-world existence. Cancer has been my underworld summons, but it is only one of many experiences that may tear open a life and beckon or even force one to come to terms with a different perspective. It is a difficult journey, but one that offers an opportunity for growth and transformation.

So what are the final questions I live with after cancer? Have I learned enough? Have I done enough? Have I been courageous enough? Have I spoken and lived my truth? Have I loved well enough? Scary questions, to be sure. Caroline Stevens, a colleague and wise woman, told me years ago that it is simple. She used to say there are only two requirements for living a conscious and authentic life: show up and pay attention. Simple, perhaps, but maybe not easy. I have to remind myself this is a journey of becoming whole, not of being perfect.

I keep two thoughts with me as I savor each day that is gifted to me. As the psalmist says, "this is the day that the Lord has made; let us rejoice and be glad in it" (Ps. 118:24). And one of my favorite poets, E. E. Cummings, expresses the same prayerful moment of gratitude: "i thank You God for most this amazing / day."

I wonder sometimes if this kind of inner exploration would be valuable to me if cancer returns, if it would be valuable to anyone facing a terminal diagnosis. Is there a facile quality in this kind of metaphorical mining, one that is all too easy to tolerate at this distance from the terrifying reality of illness and death? Is the ultimate value dependent upon the final stage? Is the crucial goal to die with consciousness, with some measure of acceptance and peace?

That, I think, may be too narrow a view, another emphasis on product and a failure to trust and honor the process. I don't know what will be useful when I face death more intimately, but I do know my life has been deepened and enriched by the experience of breast cancer. Perhaps it is enough to stay focused in the present moment, to be grateful for the joys of the day and to continue to struggle with the challenge of being faithful to the truth of my experience, to the truth of who I am. With the tree as one of the recurring symbols of my inner work, I love the words of May Sarton's question of herself: "To what have I been faithful in the end? . . . To a gnarled tree, a root."[1]

As I offer the work of my inner exploration to others on the path, my wish is that you explore your own inner meanings, to learn to read the text of your book, to be the witness for your own underworld journey, to find your own redbud tree that calls to you. My specific images may resonate with the experiences of other women and may signal a need in our society for increased valuing of the feminine. But more important than these truths is the need to attend to and honor the imaginal realms of psyche as it speaks to each of us in unique individual manifestations, in the whispers of soul.

NOTES

Chapter 1

1. Annie Dillard, *The Annie Dillard Reader* (New York: Harper, 1994), 265.
2. C. G. Jung, "Commentary on 'The Secret of the Golden Flower,'" *Alchemical Studies*, vol. 13, *The Collected Works of C. G. Jung* (Princeton, NJ: Princeton University Press, 1967), par. 54.
3. Russell Lockhart, *Words as Eggs* (Dallas: Spring Publications, 1983), 65–66.
4. Albert Kreinheder, "The Call to Individuation," *Psychological Perspectives* 10, no. 1 (1979): 64.

Chapter 2

1. T. S. Eliot, *Four Quartets* (San Diego: Harcourt Brace Jovanovich, 1971), 15.
2. Gerard Manley Hopkins, "God's Grandeur," *Gerard Manley Hopkins: Poems and Prose*, edited by W. H. Gardner (Baltimore, MD: Penguin Books, 1953), 27.
3. Gaston Bachelard, *On Poetic Imagination and Reverie: Selections from Gaston Bachelard*, translated by C. Gaudin (Dallas: Spring Publications, 1987), 91, 79.
4. May Sarton, *Plant Dreaming Deep* (New York: W. W. Norton, 1968), p. 11.
5. Quoted in J. Maritain, *Creative Intuition in Art and Poetry* (New York: Meridian Books, 1953), 110.
6. Russell Lockhart, *Words as Eggs* (Dallas: Spring Publications, 1983), 212.
7. Rainer Maria Rilke, *Letters to a Young Poet* (New York: W. W. Norton, 1954), 35.
8. Wallace Stevens, *The Collected Poems of Wallace Stevens* (New York: Alfred A. Knopf, 1961), 94.
9. Rainer Maria Rilke, *Selected Poems of Rainer Maria Rilke*, translated by Robert Bly (New York: Harper and Row, 1981), 13.
10. Bachelard, *On Poetic Imagination and Reverie*, 94, 83.
11. Ibid., 97.
12. "Ars Poetica," quoted in G. D. Sanders, J. H. Nelson, and M. L. Rosenthal, eds., *Chief Modern Poets of England and America* (New York: Macmillan, 1962), 334.

13. James Hillman, *Re-visioning Psychology* (New York: Harper and Row, 1975), 39.

Chapter 3

1. James Hillman, *The Myth of Analysis* (New York: Harper, 1978), 283.
2. Alice Koller, *An Unknown Woman* (New York: Bantam, 1983), 78.
3. Kim Chernin, *Reinventing Eve* (New York: Harper, 1987), 15.
4. Ibid., xiii, xv.
5. Marion Woodman, *The Pregnant Virgin* (Toronto: Inner City Books, 1985), 20.
6. Ibid., 22.
7. Alix Shulman, *Drinking the Rain* (New York: Penguin Books, 1996), 130.
8. Ibid., 17.
9. Ibid., 52–53.

Chapter 4

1. Judith Duerk, *Circle of Stones* (San Diego: Lura Media, 1989), 42.
2. Alice Walker, "Oppressed Hair Puts a Ceiling on the Brain," *Living by the Word: Selected Writings 1973–1987* (Orlando, FL: Harcourt, Brace, Jovanovich, 1988, pp. 69–74), 71.
3. Ibid., 72–73.
4. C. G. Jung, *Psychological Types*, vol. 6, *The Collected Works of C. G. Jung* (Princeton, NJ: Princeton University Press, 1971), par. 723.
5. T. S. Eliot, *Four Quartets* (San Diego: Harcourt Brace Jovanovich, 1971), 28.

Chapter 5

1. Robert Frost, "The Secret Sits," *The Poetry of Robert Frost,* edited by E. C. Lathem (New York: Holt, Rinehart, and Winston, 1979), 362.

Chapter 6

1. Mary Watkins, *Waking Dreams* (Dallas: Spring, 1984), 20.
2. Ibid., 26
3. Lorrie Moore, *Anagrams* (New York: Penguin, 1986), 36.
4. Deena Metzger, *The Book of Hags*, dramatized by Everett Frost, produced for KPFK, Pacifica Radio (Los Angeles, 1976; audiocassette: Black Box, Washington, DC, 1977).
5. Audre Lorde, *The Cancer Journals* (San Francisco: aunt lute books, 1980), 18–19.
6. Ibid., 20.
7. Quoted in Lorde, *The Cancer Journals*, 21.

8. Ibid., 20.
9. Watkins, *Waking Dreams*, 134.
10. Ibid., 122.
11. Moore, *Anagrams*, 10.

Chapter 7

1. Frederick Turner, "The Immortal Conversation: Culture as a Web of Thought" (lecture, Pacifica Graduate Institute, Santa Barbara, CA, April 7, 1990).
2. Ibid.
3. Quoted in *When I Am an Old Woman I Shall Wear Purple*, edited by Sandra Haldeman Martz (Manhattan Beach, CA: Papier-Mache Press, 1987), 73.
4. Erich Fromm, *To Have or To Be?* (New York: Bantam, 1976), 14.
5. Ibid., 22.
6. Ibid., 39.
7. Ibid., 40.
8. Ibid., 49.
9. Ibid., 96.
10. Ibid., 97.
11. Quoted in Laurie Lisle, *Portrait of an Artist: A Biography of Georgia O'Keeffe* (New York: Washington Square Press, 1981), 295.
12. Thich Nhat Hanh, *Peace Is Every Step* (New York: Bantam, 1991), 95.
13. Ibid., 96–97.
14. May Sarton, *Journal of a Solitude* (New York: W. W. Norton, 1973), 201.

Chapter 8

1. Quoted in Alix Shulman, *Drinking the Rain* (New York: Penguin Books, 1996), 206.
2. Anne Sexton, *The Complete Poems* (Boston: Houghton Mifflin, 1981), 94.
3. Clarissa Pinkola Estés, *Women Who Run with the Wolves* (New York: Random House, 1992), 66.
4. Ibid., 66.
5. C. P. Cavafy, *Collected Poems* (Princeton, NJ: Princeton University Press, 1975), 35–36.

Final Thoughts

1. May Sarton, *Halfway to Silence* (New York: W. W. Norton, 1980), 56.

BIBLIOGRAPHY

Bachelard, G. *On Poetic Imagination and Reverie: Selections from Gaston Bachelard.* C. Gaudin, trans. Dallas: Spring Publications, 1987.

Cavafy, C. P. *Collected Poems.* Princeton, NJ: Princeton University Press, 1975.

Chernin, Kim. *Reinventing Eve.* New York: Harper, 1987.

Craighead, Meinrad. *The Litany of the Great River.* Mahwah, NJ: Paulist Press, 1991.

Dillard, Annie. *The Annie Dillard Reader.* New York: Harper, 1994.

Duerk, Judith. *Circle of Stones.* San Diego: Lura Media, 1989.

Eliot, T. S. *Four Quartets.* San Diego: Harcourt Brace Jovanovich, 1971.

Frank, Arthur. *At the Will of the Body: Reflections on Illness.* New York: Mariner Books, 2002.

Fromm, Erich. *To Have or To Be?* New York: Bantam, 1976.

Frost, Robert. *The Poetry of Robert Frost.* E. C. Lathem, ed. New York: Holt, Rinehart, and Winston, 1979.

Hillman, James. *Re-visioning Psychology.* New York: Harper and Row, 1975.

———. *The Myth of Analysis.* New York: Harper and Row, 1978.

Hopkins, Gerard Manley. *Gerard Manley Hopkins: Poems and Prose.* W. H. Gardner, ed. Baltimore: Penguin Books, 1953.

Jones, W. Paul. *A Table in the Desert: Making Space Holy.* Brewster, MA: Paraclete Press, 2001.

Jung, C. G. "Commentary on 'The Secret of the Golden Flower,'" *Alchemical Studies*, vol. 13, *The Collected Works of C. G. Jung.* Princeton, NJ: Princeton University Press, 1967.

———. *Psychological Types*, vol. 6, *The Collected Works of C. G. Jung.* Princeton, NJ: Princeton University Press, 1971.

Koller, Alice. *An Unknown Woman.* New York: Bantam, 1983.

Kreinheder, Albert. "The Call to Individuation," *Psychological Perspectives* 10, no. 1 (1979): 58–65.

Lisle, Laurie. *Portrait of an Artist: A Biography of Georgia O'Keeffe.* New York: Washington Square Press, 1981.

Lockhart, Russell. *Words as Eggs.* Dallas: Spring Publications, 1983.

Lorde, Audre. *The Cancer Journals.* San Francisco: aunt lute books, 1980.

Maritain, J. *Creative Intuition in Art and Poetry.* New York: Meridian Books, 1953.

Martz, Sandra Haldeman, ed. *When I Am an Old Woman I Shall Wear Purple.* Manhattan Beach, CA: Papier-Mache Press, 1987.

Metzger, Deena. *The Book of Hags.* Dramatized by Everett Frost, produced for KPFK, Pacifica Radio, Los Angeles, 1976. Audiocassette: Washington, DC: Black Box, 1977.

———. *Tree: Essays and Pieces.* Berkeley, CA: North Atlantic Books, 1978.

Moore, Lorrie. *Anagrams.* New York: Penguin, 1986.

Nhat Hanh, Thich. *Peace Is Every Step.* New York: Bantam, 1991.

O'Donohue, John. *Anam Cara: A Book of Celtic Wisdom.* New York: HarperCollins, 1997.

Oliver, Mary. *Thirst.* Boston: Beacon Press, 2006.

———. *West Wind: Poems and Prose Poems.* New York: Houghton Mifflin, 1997.

Rilke, Rainer Maria. *Letters to a Young Poet.* New York: W. W. Norton, 1954.

———. *Selected Poems of Rainer Maria Rilke.* Robert Bly, trans. New York: Harper and Row, 1981.

Sanders, G. D., J. H. Nelson, and M. L. Rosenthal, eds. *Chief Modern Poets of England and America.* New York: Macmillan, 1962.

Sarton, May. *Halfway to Silence.* New York: W. W. Norton, 1980.

———. *Journal of a Solitude.* New York: W. W. Norton, 1973.

———. *Plant Dreaming Deep.* New York: W. W. Norton, 1968.

Scott, Whitney, ed. *Words Against the Shifting Seasons: Women Speak of Breast Cancer.* Limited edition, privately published.

Sexton, Anne. *The Complete Poems.* Boston: Houghton Mifflin, 1981.

Shulman, Alix. *Drinking the Rain.* New York: Penguin Books, 1996.

Stevens, Wallace. *The Collected Poems of Wallace Stevens.* New York: Alfred A. Knopf, 1961.

Walker, Alice. "Oppressed Hair Puts a Ceiling on the Brain." *Living by the Word: Selected Writings 1973–1987.* Orlando, FL: Harcourt, Brace, Jovanovich, 1988, 69–74.

Watkins, Mary. *Waking Dreams.* Dallas: Spring, 1984.

Woodman, Marion. *The Pregnant Virgin.* Toronto: Inner City Books, 1985.

INDEX